PHILIP W. LEBOWITZ

Handbook of Epidural Anaesthesia and Analgesia

Handbook of Epidural Anaesthesia and Analgesia

BENJAMIN G. COVINO
PH.D., M.D.

Chairman, Department of Anesthesia
Brigham and Women's Hospital
Professor of Anesthesia
Harvard Medical School
Boston, Mass. USA

D.BRUCE SCOTT
M.D., F.R.C.P.E., F.F.A.R.C.S.

Consultant Anaesthetist, Royal Infirmary; and, Senior Lecturer, Department of Anaesthetics, University of Edinburgh, Edinburgh, Scotland

LENNART HÅKANSSON

Coordinator

POUL BUCKHÖJ

Medical artist

KARSTEN HJERTHOLM

Photo

POUL BUCKHÖJ

Layout

G&S

GRUNE & STRATTON, INC.
(Harcourt Brace Jovanovich, Publishers)
Orlando San Diego New York
London Toronto Montreal Sydney Tokyo

21, Møntergade
DK-1116 Copenhagen K
Denmark
Printed by J. H. Schultz A/S, 1985

United States Edition Published by
GRUNE & STRATTON, INC.
Orlando, Florida 32887

ISBN (Schultz) 87-569-1180-7

ISBN (G&S) 0-8089-1742-0

Foreword

Over 61 years ago the master surgeon William J. Mayo in his foreword to Gaston Labat's classic volume "Regional Anesthesesia" wrote that "regional anesthesia has come to stay". Not only has it stayed but its popularity has steadily increased among anaesthetists surgeons and patients, especially since the introduction of the amide-linked drugs 35 years ago. Epidural anaesthesia in surgery, obstetrics and in the relief of acute pain is now one of the most frequently used techniques of regional analgesia and arouses worldwide interest. Thus it is important that anaesthetists should have available authoritative texts to consult which enable them to share the accumulated theoretical and practical knowledge of workers of great experience, and from the information so gained can put into practice in a safe and satisfactory manner, what they have learnt.

Correlation of accumulated facts and theories becomes an important service in these days of rapid change and development in our specialty. This book condenses the lessons of the authors' vast and varied experience, gained as teachers, investigators and clinical anaesthetists in Britain and in the U.S. This symbiotic double authorship will make the text acceptable to anaesthetists adhering to both Anglo-Saxon and North American traditions.

There are several aspects that make it a valuable, interesting and welcome addition to the currently available works on epidural anaesthesia. One of these is the large number of informative, interesting and beautiful illustrations in full colour. Another is the section devoted to the use of epidural opioids. Perhaps even more importantly it informs the reader in a straightforward manner hcw to administer an epidural block and how to manage the patient afterwards.

The authors have succeeded in laying before the reader a clear yet detailed description of the best methods of inducing, maintaining and monitoring epidural anaesthesia during the operation or delivery. The prevention and management of any complications which may arise are not neglected. It is a book to which reference may be made should any problems connected with epidural anaesthesia cause concern. It is the type of book which will enable an anaesthetist, by referring to its pages, to obtain practical advice which will materially assist him in the management and conduct of the case.

The value of epidural block increases with the degree of skill with which it is administered, and reading this book and following its teaching will enable that skill to be achieved, if the precepts it contains are followed.

The object in writing this monograph was to produce an authoritative and clearly written text in which the reader can easily find the information he desires, and the authors have succeeded admirably in this praiseworthy task.

J. Alfred Lee

Preface

The primary purpose in writing this book was to produce a well illustrated text which provides the basic information required by the average anaesthetist, who occasionally uses epidural anaesthesia and, in particular, anaesthetists-in-training who should be encouraged to learn the technique. We have been very fortunate to obtain the services of the artist, Poul Buckhöj, whose work will be familiar to those who perform regional anaesthesia. Since we feel that drawings and photographs of high quality are preferable to the written word in terms of describing a technique which requires a knowledge of anatomy, the book has been intentionally heavily illustrated and the written text kept brief but hopefully clear in its meaning.

As indicated by the title, the book is intended to be essentially practical in nature and not an exhaustive treatise on epidural blockade. There already exist several excellent texts, which provide in depth reference sources for the individual who is interested in a more exhaustive review of this topic. Little purpose would have been served to simply duplicate these efforts. Nevertheless, we have attempted to cover the major issues concerning epidural anaesthesia and provide, we trust, a balanced view of the controversies which exist in this field and await elucidation. Thus, for example, we have reviewed the advantages of this technique as compared to general anaesthesia but have also attempted to present the potential hazards and problems associated with epidural anaesthesia. The anatomy, physiology and pharmacology of epidural anaesthesia and analgesia have been described since a knowledge of these areas is essential in order to derive the greatest benefits from this anaesthetic technique. Since the text was intended to be a practical handbook, we have made no attempt to reference all of the statements but instead have provided what we believe to be the pertinent references at the conclusion of each chapter. The interested reader is encouraged to investigate those references which serve as the scientific base for the statements made in the text.

There are considerable problems facing two authors separated by the Atlantic Ocean. We trust we have largely overcome the difficulties, but in any case, we remain the best of friends which is a significant fact in itself. We have used English idioms and spelling, rather than American, throughout. In the text drug names are given in the World Health Organization's International Non-proprietary Name (I.N.N.) convention, and a list of generic and trade names are on p. 170. Because practice varies from country to country and may indeed have legal implications, we have tried not to be too dogmatic in regard to some of the clinical aspects such as monitoring, aseptic technique etc. Anaesthetists should have no trouble in modifying our recommendations to suit their local circumstances.

Many individuals assisted in the preparation of this text. In particular, we wish to express our great debt to Lennart Håkansson of ICM AB, who kept us firmly at our task and was quite essential in the whole endeavour. In addition, we want to thank Ms. Bonnie Brugger and Lorna Robertson for the many revisions of the text which required their typing expertise. Finally, we wish to acknowledge our respective spouses, Joan Scott and Lorraine Covino, for their patience and understanding of the many hours that were spent in this task.

Benjamin G. Covino and D. Bruce Scott

Contents

1. Anatomical considerations

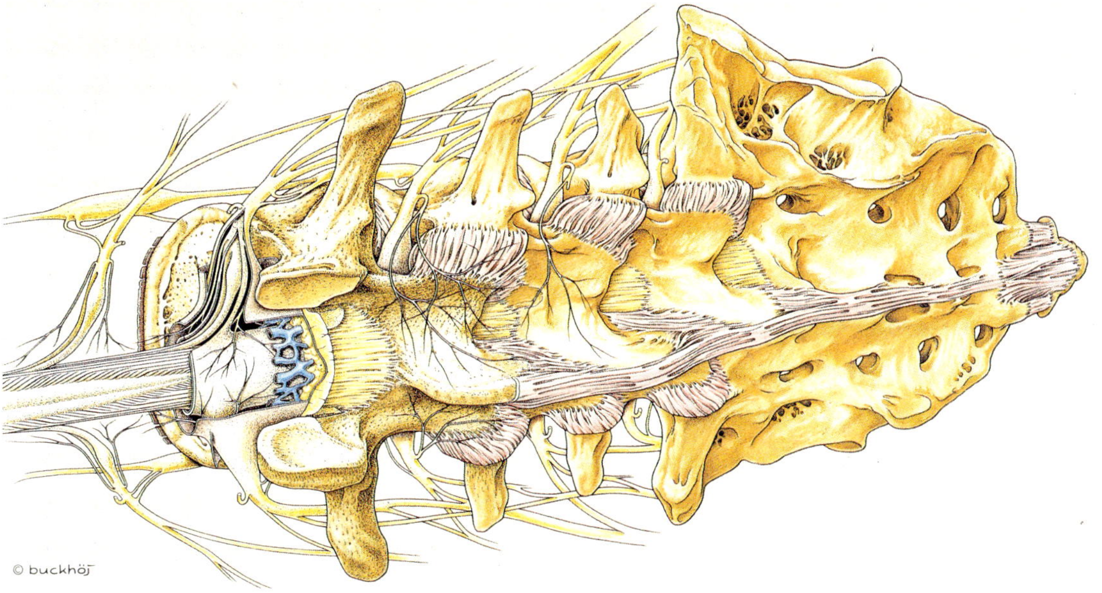

© buckhöj

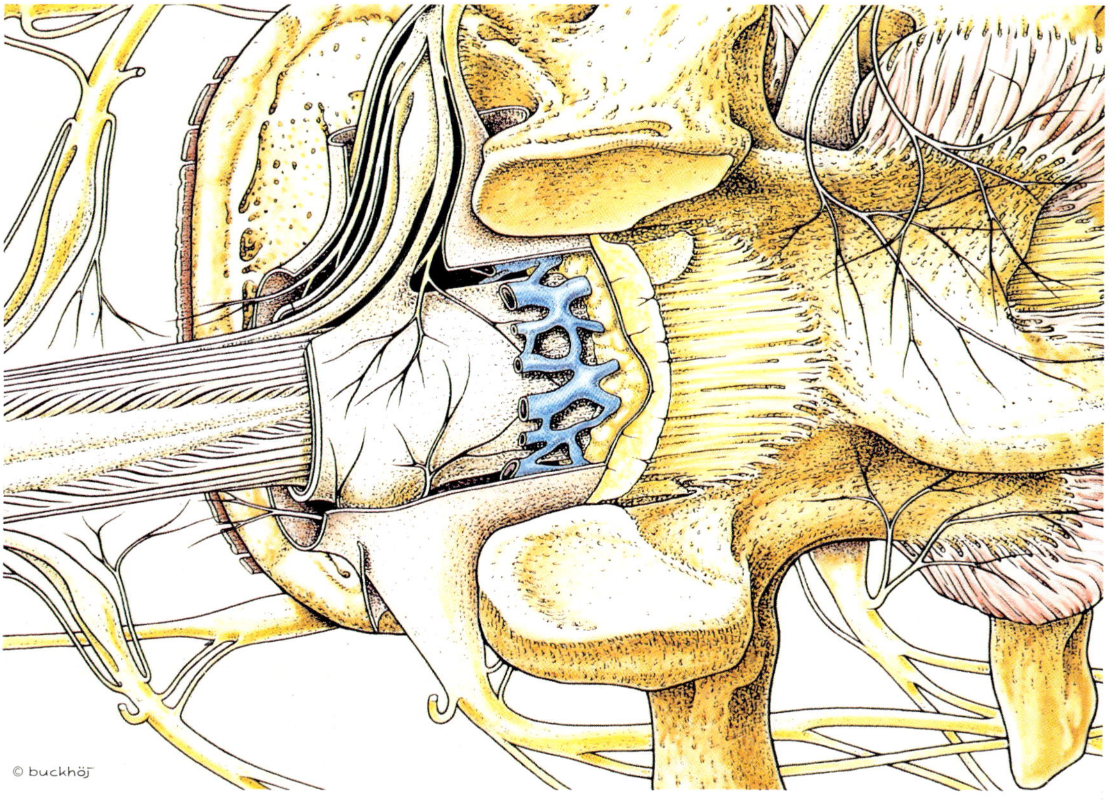

© buckhöj

Vertebral column

Since epidural anaesthesia requires the injection of local anaesthetic drugs into the extradural space within the spinal canal, a proper understanding of the anatomy is essential. The canal runs from the foramen magnum to the sacral hiatus (Fig. 1:1). The bony arches of the vertebrae posterior to the vertebral bodies form a continuum to make up the spinal canal, the spaces between the vertebrae being taken up by the spinal ligaments.

The vertebral column is composed of 7 cervical, 12 thoracic and 5 lumbar vertebrae, with the sacrum and coccyx inferiorly (Fig. 1:2). Though all the vertebrae have a common structure, they vary in shape and size according to their position and function. The cervical vertebrae, having the least weight bearing and the maximum amount of movement, are relatively small compared with the large robust vertebrae in the lumbar region.

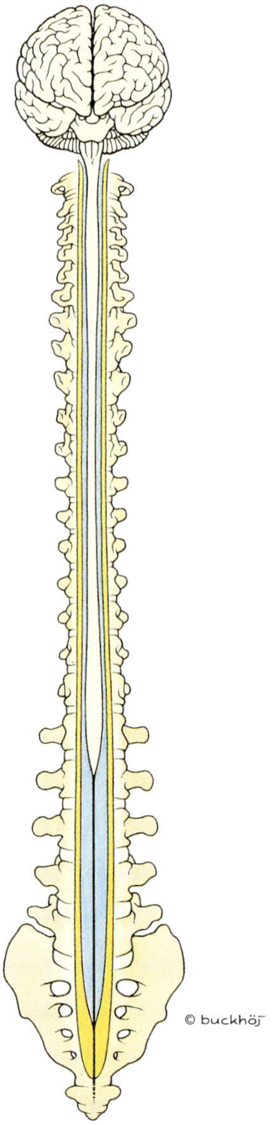

Fig. 1:1

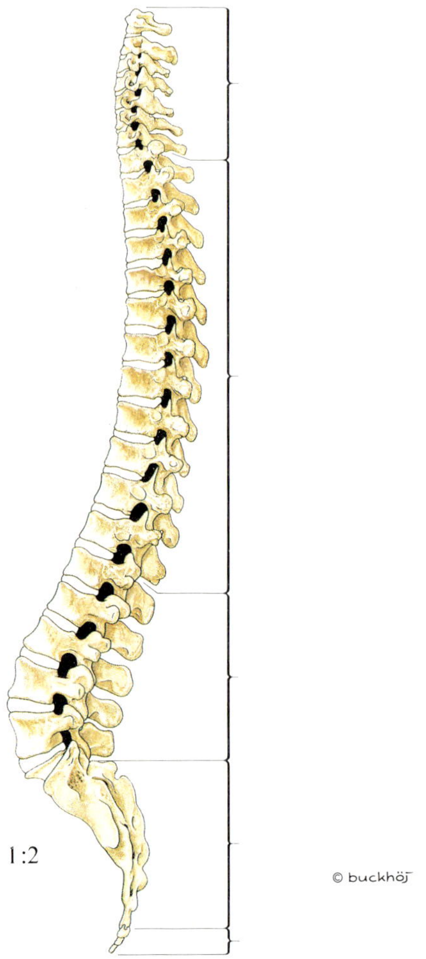

Fig. 1:2

A vertebra is made up of a vertebral body behind which is a bony arch (Fig. 1:3). The arch consists of two pedicles anteriorly and two laminae posteriorly. At the junction of pedicles and laminae are the transverse processes. Where the laminae meet is the spinous process.

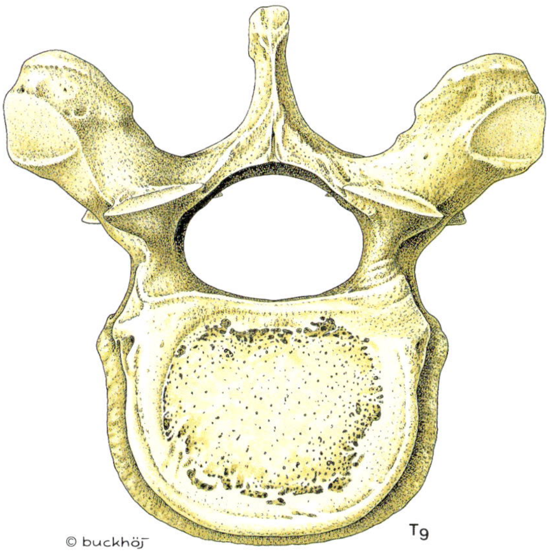

Fig. 1:3 Typical thoracic vertebra.

The spinous processes vary in regard to their angulation (Fig. 1:4). This is important in attempting to locate the epidural space with a needle.

In the cervical, lower thoracic and lumbar region the processes are almost horizontal and a needle may be inserted at right angles to the sagittal plane.

In the mid-thoracic region the spinous processes are directed caudally and this angulation becomes maximal between T_3 and T_7, thus requiring the needle to be inserted at varying degrees from the horizontal.

Fig. 1:4 Oblique views of a cervical, a thoracic and a lumbar vertebra.

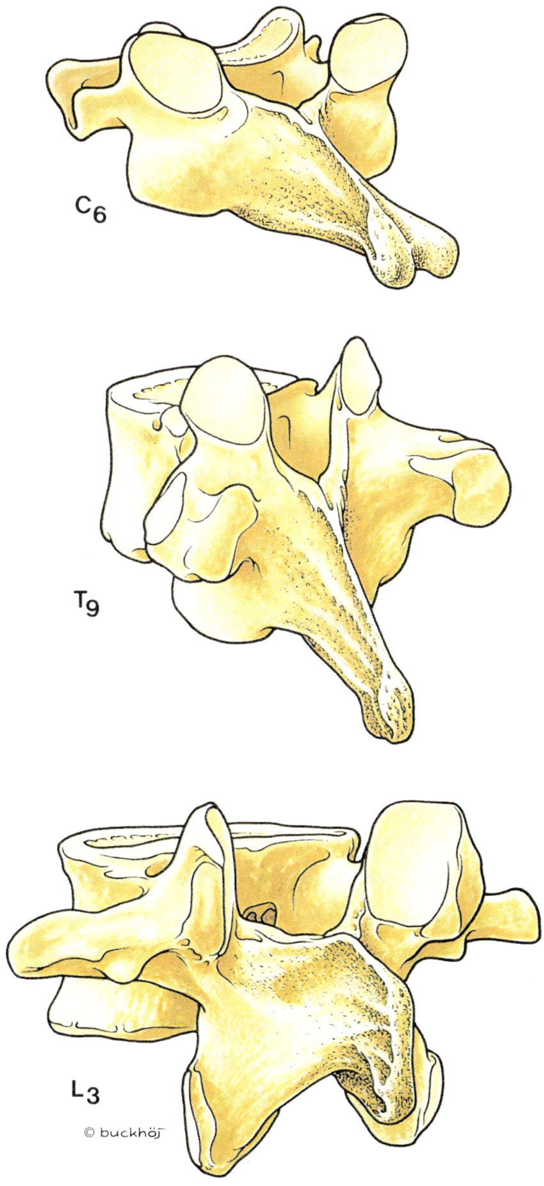

The sacrum is formed by the fusion of the 5 sacral vertebrae inside which the spinal canal continues its downward progress to end at the sacral hiatus, which is a gap in the fifth sacral vertebra due to the absence of its laminae (Fig. 1:5a and b).

Occasionally the laminae of S_4 and even S_3 are also absent, causing an abnormally large hiatus.

The coccyx is attached to the sacrum inferiorly.

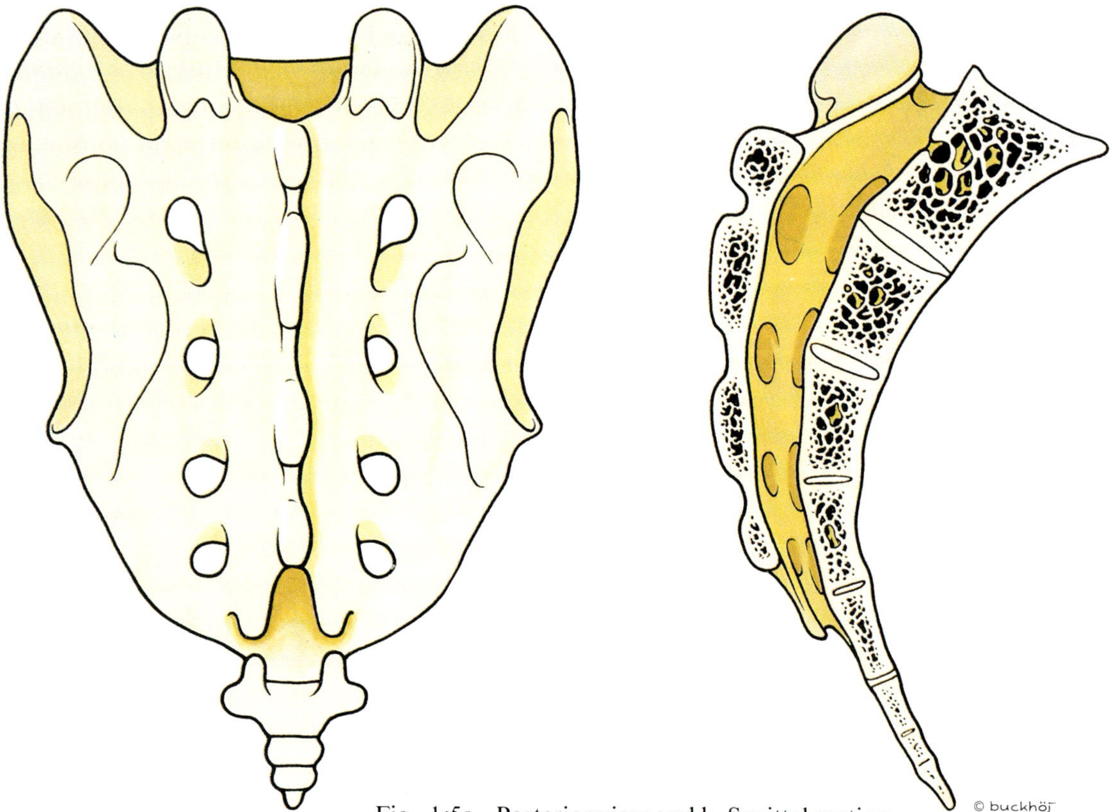

Fig. 1:5a. Posterior view and b. Sagittal section of the sacrum and coccyx.

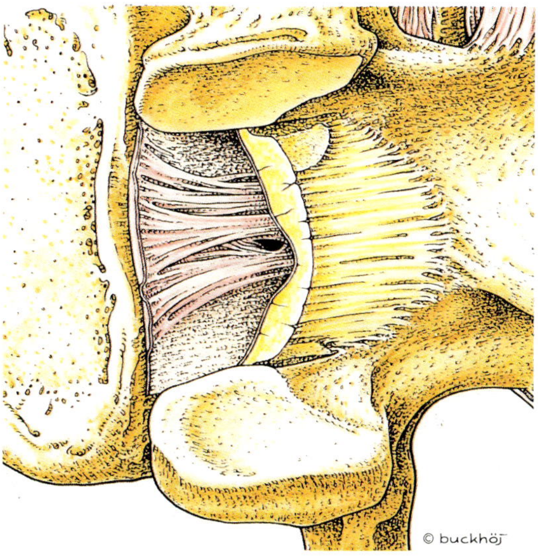

Fig. 1:6 Posterior view of the second and third lumbar vertebrae showing the attachment of the spinal ligaments.

Spinal ligaments

Adjacent vertebrae are held together posteriorly by short tough ligaments and it is through these ligaments that access to the spinal canal is achieved (Figs. 1:6 and 1:7). The laminae of the vertebrae are connected by the ligamentum flavum while the posterior spinous processes are connected by the interspinous ligament. The supraspinous ligament runs superficial to the tips of the spinous processes. Anteriorly the bodies of the vertebrae are separated by the intervertebral discs and the anterior longitudinal ligament runs from the skull to the sacrum with firm attachments to the discs and the adjacent margins of the vertebral bodies. The posterior longitudinal ligament connects the posterior aspects of the vertebral bodies and forms the anterior wall of the vertebral canal.

The pedicles are not connected by ligaments. The resulting aperture, the intervertebral foramen, is necessary to allow the spinal nerves to leave the spinal canal.

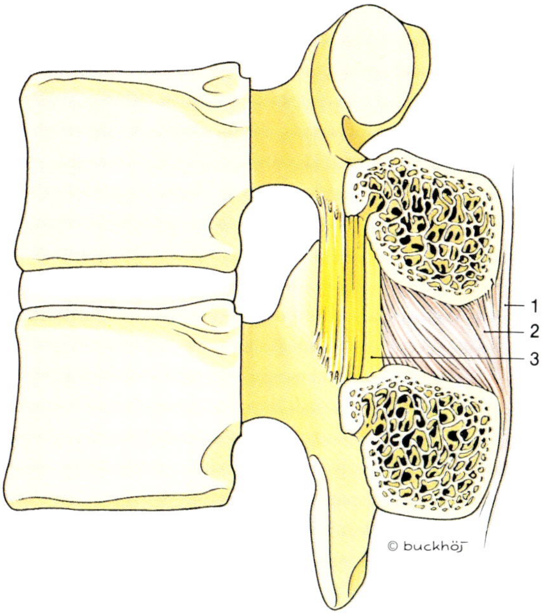

Fig. 1:7 Sagittal section through the second and third lumbar vertebrae showing the ligaments attached to the adjacent laminae and spinous process.

1. Supraspinous ligament
2. Interspinous ligament
3. Ligamentum flavum

To insert a needle into the spinal canal between two vertebrae, it must traverse the supraspinous and intraspinous ligaments before reaching the ligamentum flavum, the last barrier to the canal itself.

The ligamentum flavum is tougher than the others and it is usually easy to identify by its increased resistance to the needle. It is thinnest in the midline getting thicker laterally. Its function is to hold adjacent laminae firmly together and it forms, together with the laminae, the posterior wall of the spinal canal.

The attachments of the ligamentum flavum extend laterally to the articular capsules (Fig. 1:8). It is firmly connected to the lower anterior border of the lamina above and the upper margin of the lamina below The ligamentum flavum varies in size and shape at different levels of the vertebral column (Fig. 1:9).

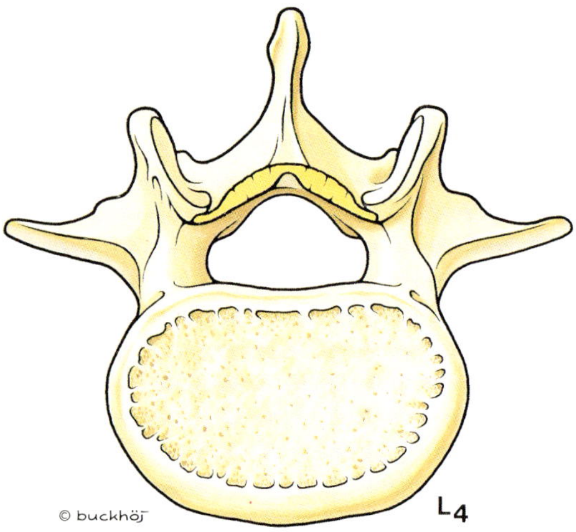

Fig. 1:8 Superior view of a lumbar vertebra showing the attachment of the ligamentum flavum.

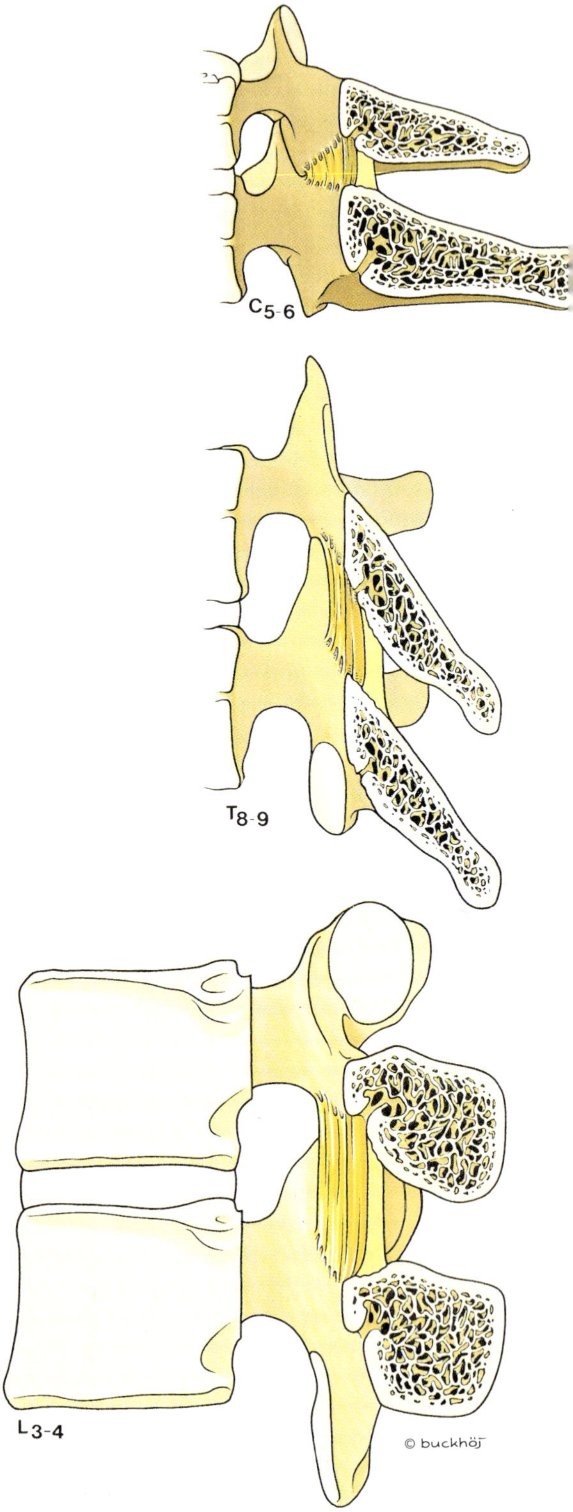

Fig. 1:9 Ligamenta flavae in a. Cervical spine. b. Thoracic spine. and c. Lumbar spine.

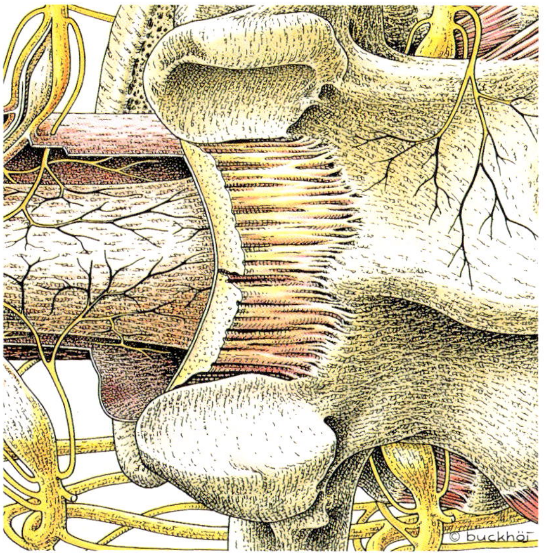

Fig. 1:10. Ligamentum flavum showing midline division through which blood vessels pass. (Courtesy of Astra).

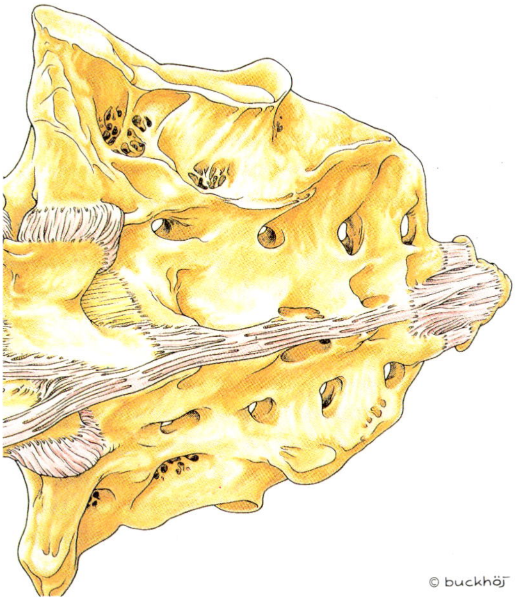

Fig. 1:11a. Oblique view and b. Sagittal section of sacrum showing the sacrococcygeal ligaments.

In some subjects the ligamentum flavum is a continuous band with no division in the midline (Fig. 1:7). In others there is such a division, through which blood vessels pass into and out of the spinal canal (Fig. 1:10). Both types of ligament can be seen at different intervertebral spaces in the same subject. These divisions account for the minimal resistance to the advancing needle occasionally encountered when performing epidural blockade.

In the sacrum there are no ligamenta flava and the laminae are all fused together, except for the fifth sacral vertebra which has no laminae and thus forms the sacral hiatus. The hiatus is covered by the sacro-coccygeal ligaments which connect the coccyx to the sacrum (Fig. 1:11a and b) .

It is through this hiatus that the spinal canal may be entered when performing a caudal (sacral) block.

Fig. 1:11b.

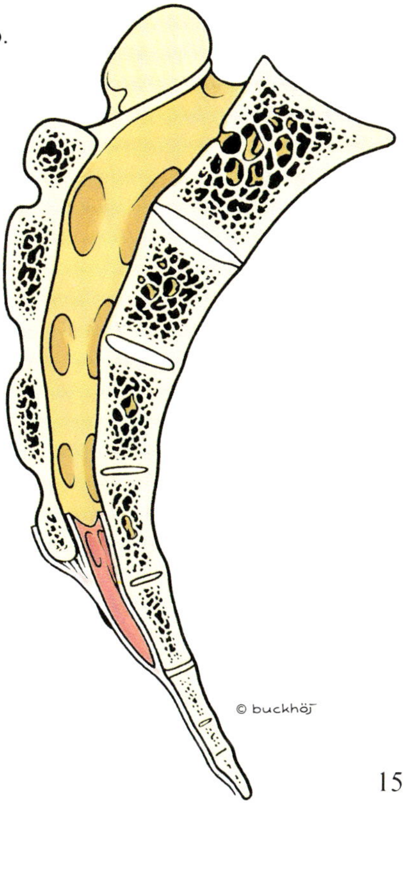

Contents of the spinal canal

The spinal canal contains the spinal cord and its three coverings, the pia mater, the arachnoid mater and the dura mater (Fig. 1:12). These create three separate spaces, the epidural space, the subdural space and the subarachnoid space. The epidural space is that part of the spinal canal outside the dura mater, enclosed by the connective tissue covering the vertebrae and the ligamentum flavum. This band of tissue, which is easily separated from the periosteum and ligamentum flavum, is referred to in older anatomy textbooks as "the outer layer of the spinal dura mater" (Fig. 1:13).

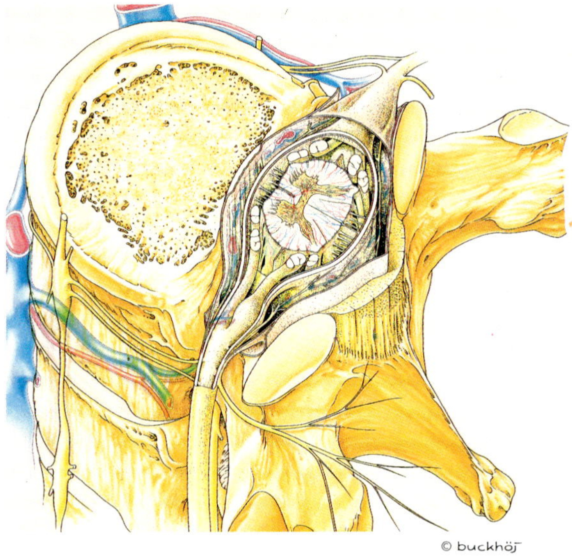

Fig. 1:12 Cross section of a thoracic vertebra showing the spinal ligaments and the contents of the dural sac.

Fig. 1:13 Cross section of the spinal canal.

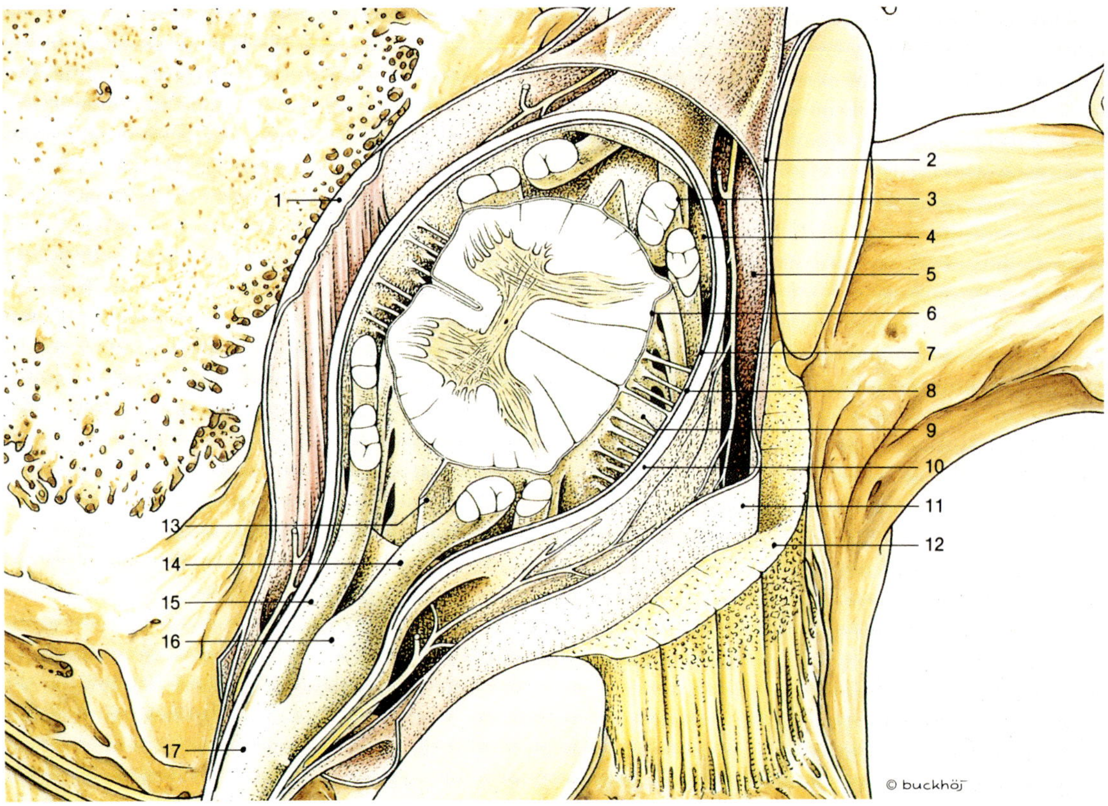

Spinal cord and its coverings

The spinal cord runs from the foramen magnum to the first or second lumbar vertebrae while the dural sac continues down to the second sacral vertebra, where it invests the filum terminale and becomes adherent to the periosteum covering the coccyx. The subdural and subarachnoid spaces thus end at the second sacral vertebra (Fig. 1:14).

1. Posterior longitudinal ligament
2. Periosteum
3. Nerve root
4. Subarachnoid space
5. Epidural space
6. Pia mater
7. Arachnoid mater
8. Subdural space
9. Subarachnoid septum
10. Dura mater (inner layer)
11. "Dura mater" (outer layer)
12. Ligamentum flavum
13. Ligamentum denticulatum
14. Dorsal nerve root
15. Ventral nerve root
16. Dorsal root ganglion
17. Spinal nerve

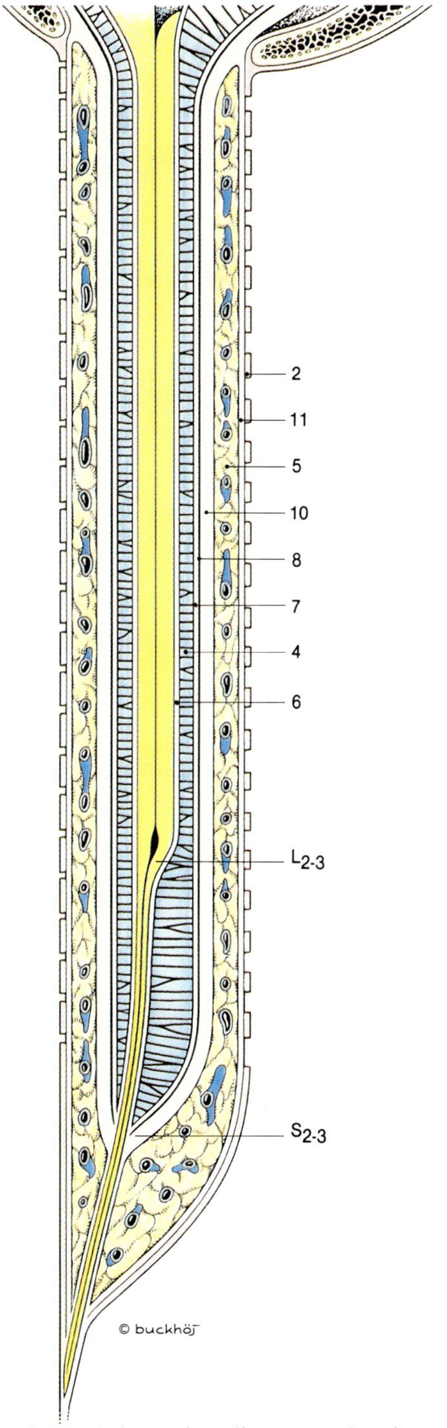

Fig. 1:14 Schematic diagram showing the levels at which the epidural space, the arachnoid space and the spinal cord terminate.

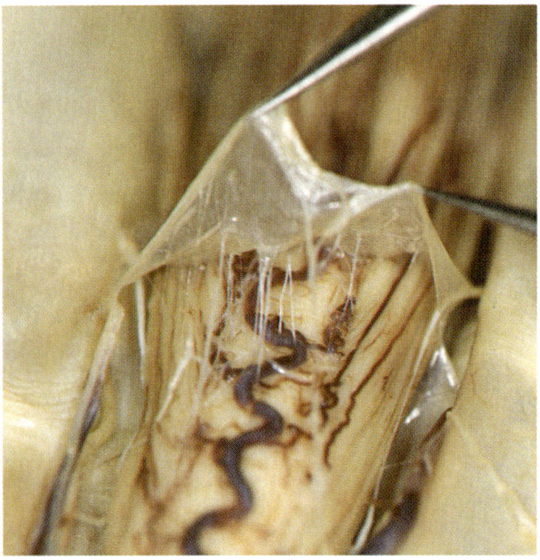

Fig. 1:15 Photograph of the spinal cord covered by the pia mater.
Photo by P. Buckhöj.

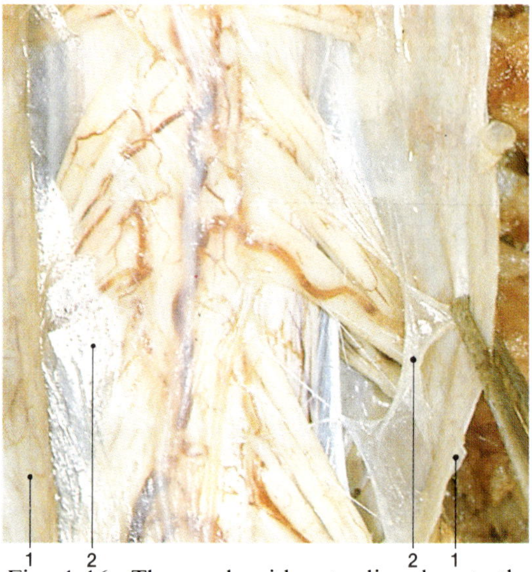

Fig. 1:16 The arachnoid mater lies close to the dura mater but they are easily separated.
Photo by P. Buckhöj.

1. Dura mater (inner layer)
2. Arachnoid mater

Pia mater

The pia mater is closely attached to the spinal cord and the spinal nerves (Fig. 1:15). Laterally it is attached to the spinal nerve roots and eventually joins the arachnoid and dura maters to become the connective tissue surrounding and investing the spinal nerves. It is separated from the arachnoid mater by the subarachnoid space containing the cerebrospinal fluid. This fluid is produced by the choroid plexuses in the brain ventricles and slowly circulates before being absorbed by the arachnoid villi.

Arachnoid mater

The arachnoid mater is a thin membrane lying close to the dura mater but easily separated from it (Fig. 1:16). The gap between the arachnoid and the dura mater is the subdural space, which is only a potential space containing lymph.

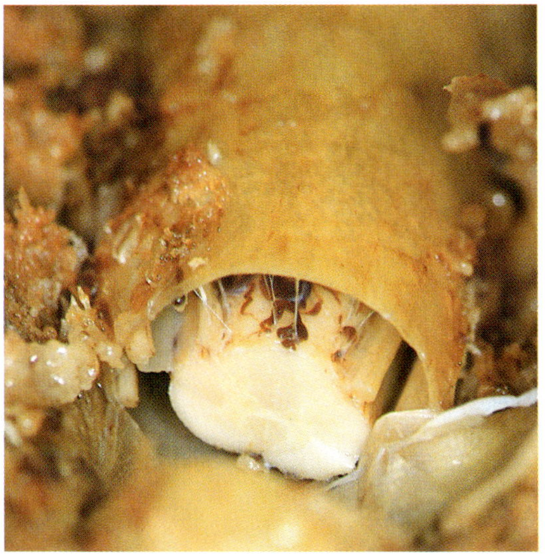

Fig. 1:17a. Photograph showing a cross section of the dural sac and its contents.
Photo by P. Buckhöj.

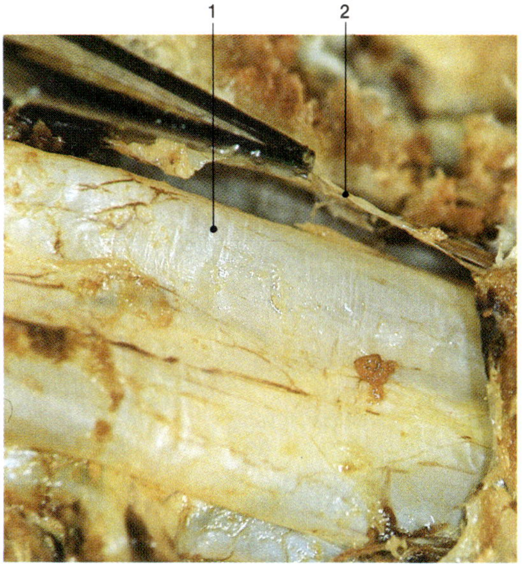

Fig. 1:17b. Photograph of the dural sac and the connective tissue layer lining the spinal canal (the "outer layer of the spinal dura") which is easily separated from bone and ligament.
Photo by P. Buckhöj.

1. Dura mater (inner layer)
2. "Dura mater" (outer layer)

Dura mater

The spinal dura mater is a thick band of tissue which envelopes the spinal cord and its inner two coverings (Fig. 1:17a and b).

As has been mentioned, older textbooks refer to this as the "inner layer of the spinal dura". At each intervertebral space a cuff of dura runs laterally with the spinal nerve and becomes adherent with the pia and arachnoid mater, and with the "outer layer of spinal dura" i.e. the connective tissue covering the vertebrae and ligaments which make up the walls of the spinal canal.

The lateral extensions of the dura, arachnoid and pia mater thus form the connective tissue covering investing the spinal nerves, i.e., the epineurium and the perineurium.

In some animal species, particularly quadrupeds, the arachnoid mater and dura mater are pierced by blood vessels supplying arachnoid granulations which are in close relationship to epidural veins (Fig. 1:18a and b). These are thought to have a similar function to the arachnoid villi in the brain and to be of importance in the circulation of cerebrospinal fluid and the transfer of drugs into, and out of, the subarachnoid space. Their presence and importance in man are disputed, however. They are frequently not present at all or exist only in small numbers in a few dural cuffs. When seen, they are close to the fusion of the arachnoid and the dura mater in the spinal nerve cuff where the epineurium is formed.

Blood supply of the spinal cord and spinal canal

Throughout the epidural space, blood vessels are numerous. These vessels supply and drain blood from the vertebrae, the spinal cord, its coverings and the spinal nerves.

The spinal cord is supplied with blood from the spinal branches of the vertebral, deep cervical, intercostal and lumbar arteries (Fig. 1:19). These spinal branches divide into anterior and posterior radicular arteries which travel along the nerve roots to reach the cord, and divide to form a plexus of arteries in the pia mater.

Fig. 1:18a. Dural cuff surrounding a spinal nerve. The close up (b.) shows arachnoid granulations penetrating the dura mater. While common in quadrupeds, they are only occasionally seen in man.

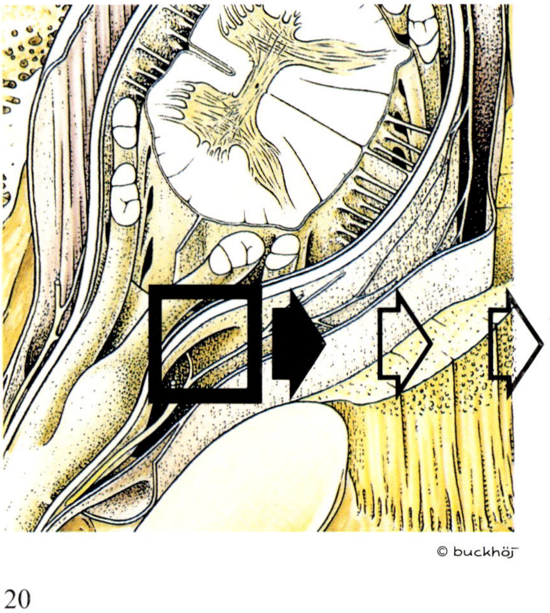

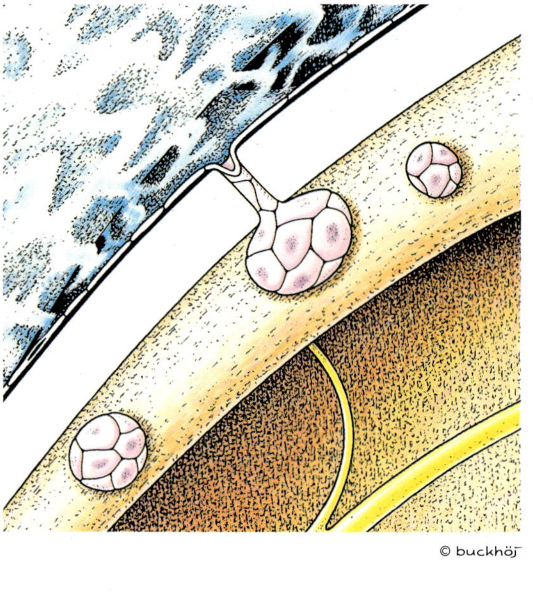

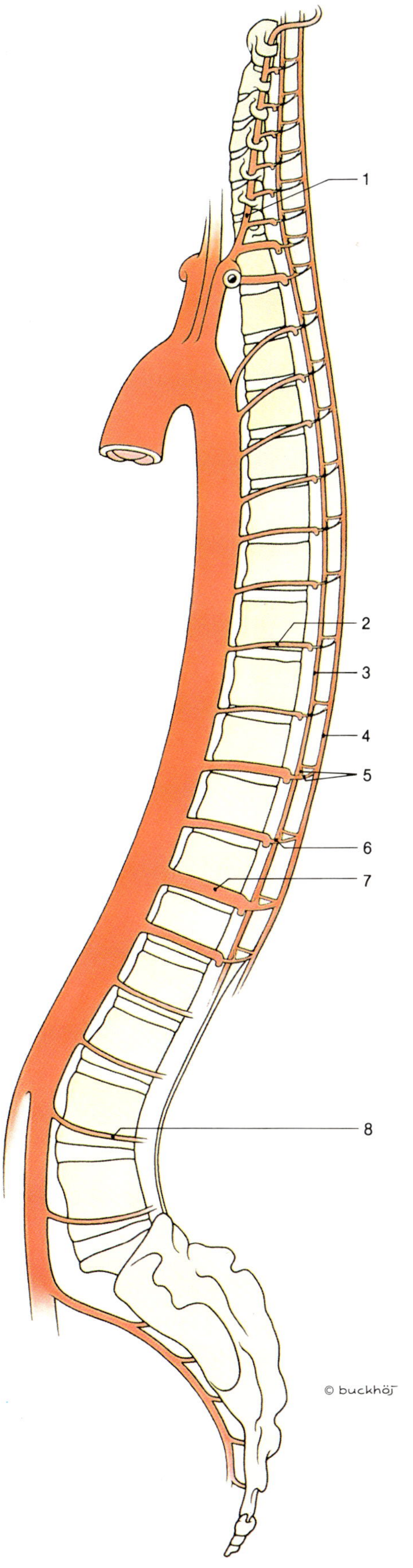

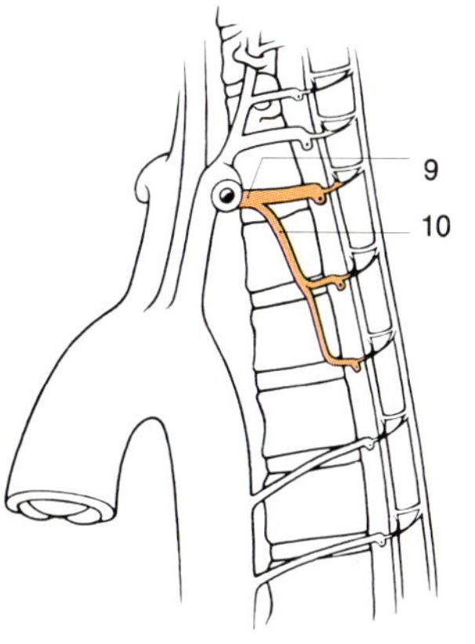

Fig. 1:19 Blood supply of the spinal cord. Radicular arteries, which run in the anterior and posterior nerve roots to the cord, are derived from the vertebral artery in the neck, the intercostal arteries in the thorax and the lumbar arteries in the abdomen. The artery of Adamkiewicz is the main supply to the lower two thirds of the cord. *Inset.* This shows the usual conformation in which the deep cervical artery gives off the radicular arteries to the eight cervical nerve roots. It then forms the superior intercostal artery supplying the first and second intercostal spaces and giving off their respective radicular arteries.

1. Vertebral artery
2. Intercostal artery
3. Anterior spinal artery
4. Posterior spinal artery
5. Anterior and posterior radicular arteries
6. Spinal branch of intercostal artery
7. Artery of Adamkiewicz
8. Lumbar artery
9. Deep cervical artery
10. Superior intercostal artery

Most of the anterior radicular branches end in the anterior nerve roots, but a variable number send superior and inferior branches which anastomose with similar arteries above and below, thus forming a single longitudinal vessel along the median sulcus of the cord, i.e., the anterior spinal artery. Usually one radicular artery is much larger than the rest and is responsible for the major part of the blood supply to the lower two-thirds of the cord. This is known as the arteria radicularis magna or the artery of Adamkiewicz, and it arises in either the lower thoracic or the upper lumbar region. It is commoner on the left side than on the right.

Posterior radicular arteries run along the posterior roots and by anastomoses above and below give rise to two posterior spinal arteries on either side of the attachment of the dorsal roots. The anterior spinal artery supplies the anterior two-thirds of the cord and the posterior spinal arteries supply the remainder, with a contribution from the plexus in the pia mater supplied by the radicular arteries. There are no anastomoses within the cord, though there is some overlap of distribution.

Blood drains into a tortuous venous plexus within the pia mater, which contains six longitudinal vessels. These connect with the internal vertebral plexus in the epidural space, which is drained via the intervertebral veins into the azygos and hemiazygos systems.

Blood from the vertebrae drains into both the internal and the external vertebral plexuses (Fig. 1:20). To reach the external plexus the veins must traverse the ligamenta flava or leave the vertebrae directly.

Spinal nerves

The anterior and posterior (dorsal) spinal nerve roots may run in separate cuffs, or a single cuff, of arachnoid and dura mater before joining to form the spinal nerves at each intervertebral space (Fig. 1:21). When they reach the intervertebral foramen, the pia, arachnoid and dura mater unite and leave the spinal canal to form the epineurium and perineurium. The epineurium covers the whole spinal nerve while the perineurium covers each bundle of nerve fibres (the funiculae) within the mixed nerve. Some authorities claim that the perineurium is derived from the lateral extension of the pia mater.

The dorsal root ganglia show considerable variation in their position. Most commonly they are just at or slightly lateral to the union of the anterior and posterior roots. Occasionally they are more lateral or more medial. Only lateral to the ganglia do the nerve fibres intermingle to form the mixed spinal nerve.

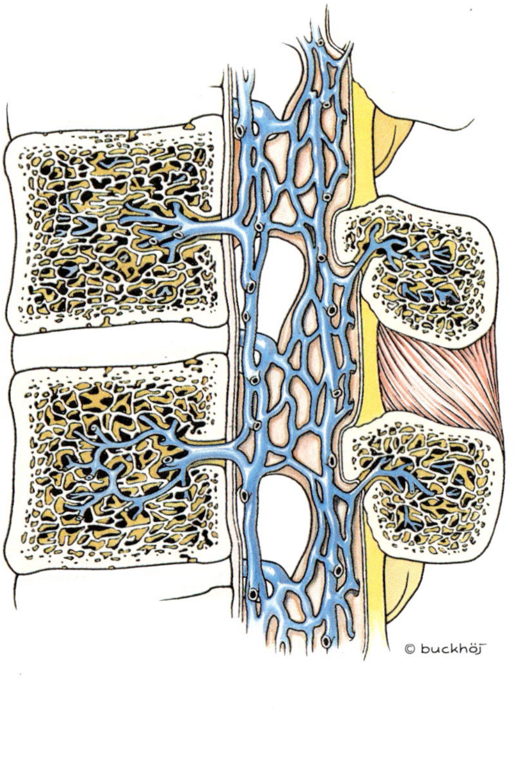

Fig. 1:20 Venous drainage of the lumbar vertebrae and spinal canal.

Fig. 1:21 Cross section of the thoracic spinal canal showing the formation of the spinal nerves by union of the anterior and posterior spinal nerve roots. Only a single nerve cuff is shown though there are frequently two cuffs, one for the anterior and one for the posterior root. The position of the dorsal root ganglion is variable (see text).

1. Arachnoid mater
2. Subdural space
3. Dura mater (inner layer)
4. "Dura mater" (outer layer)
5. Ligamentum flavum
6. Pia mater
7. Subarachnoid space
8. Epidural space
9. Dorsal root ganglion
10. Periosteum
11. Posterior longitudinal ligament

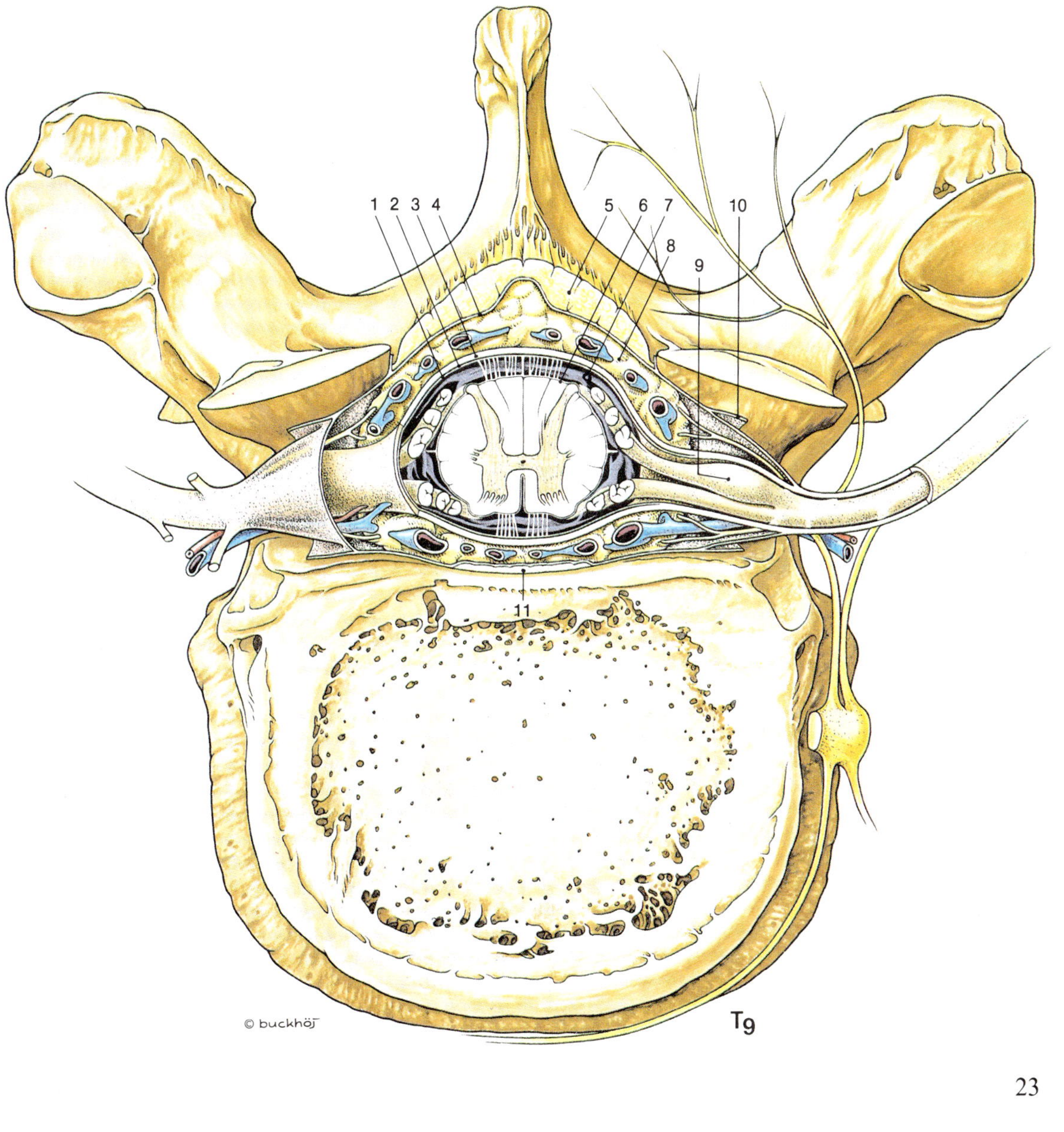

As the spinal cord ends at the level of L_{1-2}, the lower lumbar and sacral nerve roots have a long course within the spinal canal, where they form the cauda equina (Fig. 1:22). The nerves are located initially in the subarachnoid space, and then leave at the termination of the dura mater at S_1 to enter the sacral epidural space. The dorsal root ganglia of the sacral nerves may be grouped around the tip of the dural sac or may be some inches from it near the intervertebral foramina.

Although it is usual for the spinal cord to end at L_1-L_2 and the dura mater at S_2, variations do occur and these may be of clinical importance if they are lower than normal.

Fig. 1:22 Schematic diagram of the cauda equina and the formation of the lumbosacral plexus.

1. Cauda equina
2. Subarachnoid space
3. Dorsal root ganglion
4. Sacral epidural space

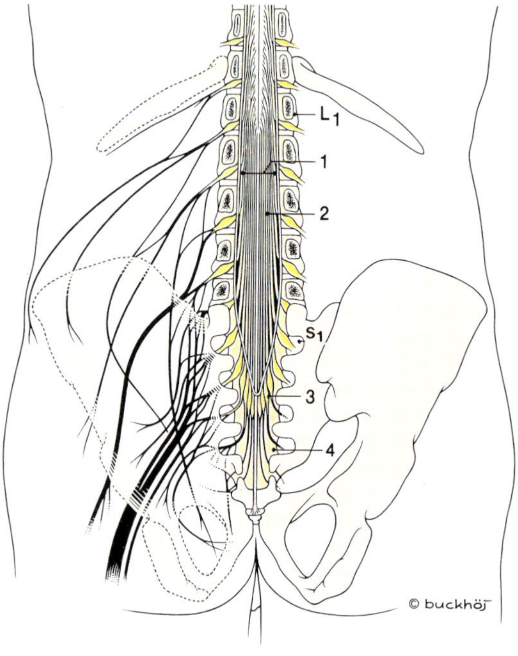

Segmental distribution of spinal nerves

The spinal nerves which leave the spinal canal through each intervertebral foramen quickly divide into anterior and posterior primary rami. The latter supply the skin and muscles of the back. The anterior rami supply the rest of the body.

Each spinal segment supplies a specific region of the skin and a specific number of muscles. In the cervical, brachial and lumbosacral regions the anterior rami join to form nerve plexuses.

In epidural blockade, motor paralysis affects the movement of various joints and muscles. The innervation of these is shown in the following list.

Shoulder	C_{6-8}
Elbow	C_{5-8}
Wrist	C_{6-7}
Hand and digits	C_{7-8}, T_1
Intercostal	T_{1-11}
Diaphragm	C_{3-5}
Abdominal	T_{7-12}
Hip, flexion	L_{1-3}
Hip, extension	L_5, S_1
Knee, flexion	L_5, S_1
Knee, extension	L_{3-4}
Ankle, flexion	L_{4-5}
Ankle, extension	S_{1-2}

The cutaneous distribution of the spinal nerves is shown in Figs. 1:23a and b. It should be remembered that there is considerable overlap between the segmental innervation of the skin. The data were originally obtained from patients with spinal nerve injuries and depended upon clinical neurological observations and not anatomical dissection. Fig. 1:23 is derived from several authorities and should be considered as a guide only.

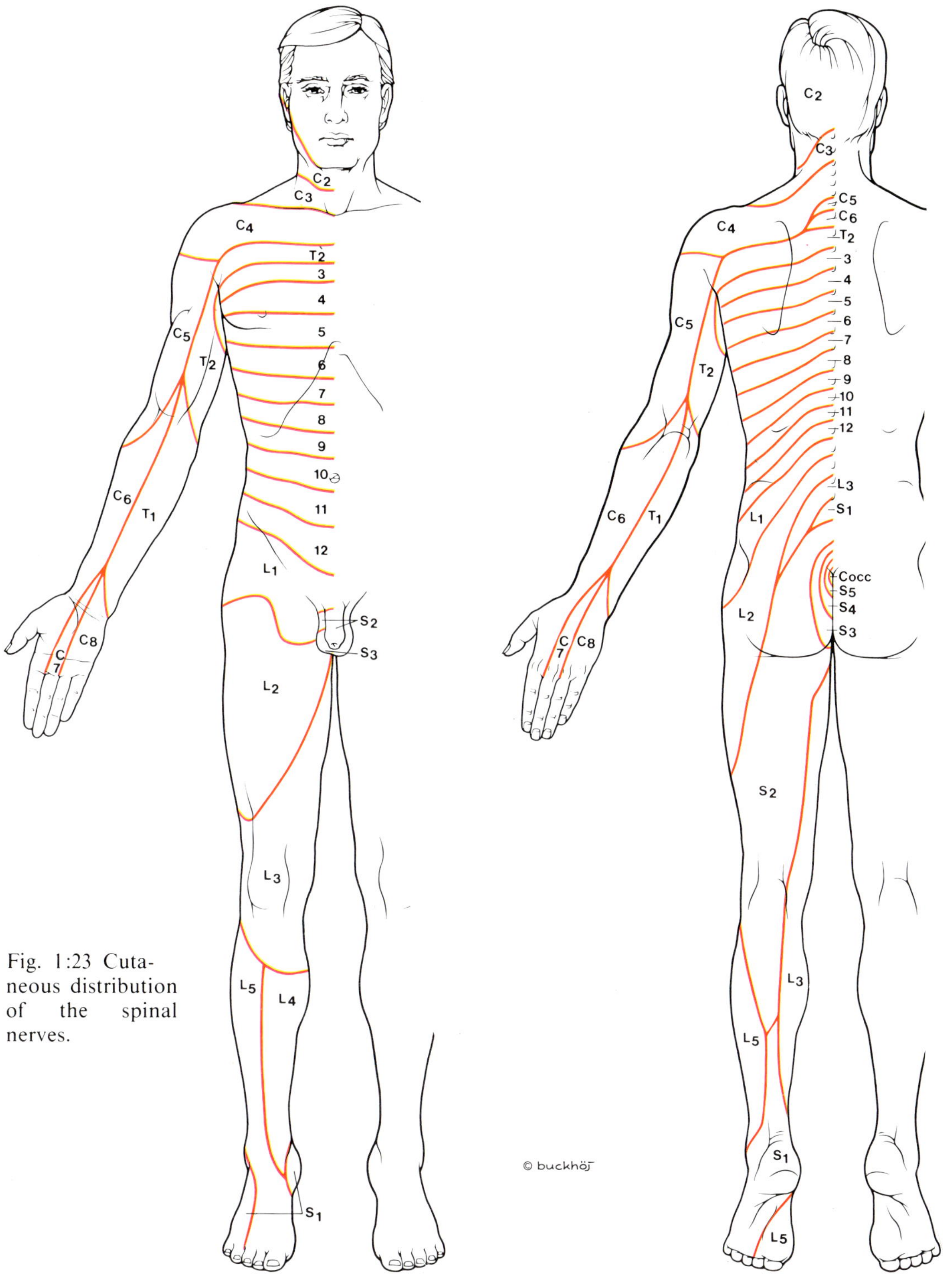

Fig. 1:23 Cutaneous distribution of the spinal nerves.

Contents of the epidural space

The epidural space contains fat and blood vessels (Fig. 1:24a and b). The fat is rather gelatinous at body temperature and is tightly packed in the space. More fat is present under the ligamenta flava and around the spinal nerves than under the bony laminae.

The epidural space is limited laterally owing to the attachment of the dura to the connective tissue covering the vertebrae and the ligamenta flava, i.e.,"the inner" and "outer" layers of the spinal dura mater fuse.

The epidural space should thus be considered as a closed compartment limited by the dura internally and by the connective tissue lining the spinal canal externally.

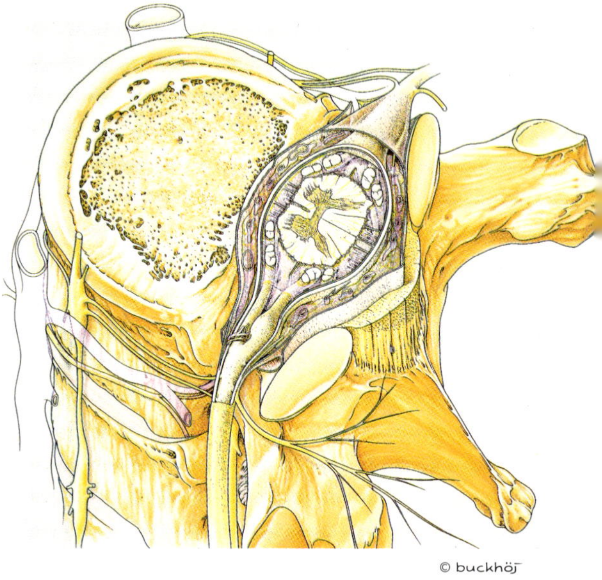

Fig. 1:24 a. and b. Oblique view of a cross section of the thoracic spine showing the contents of the epidural space.

Fig. 1:24b.

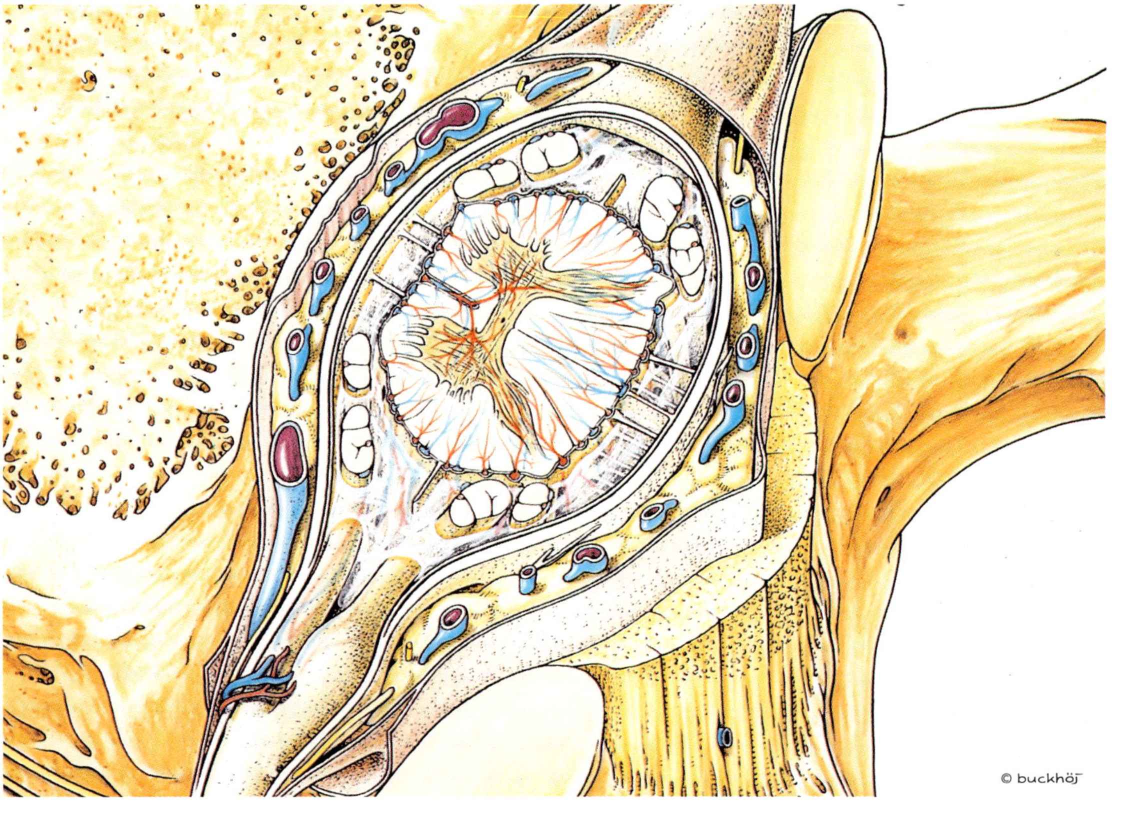

Injections of radio-opaque solutions into the epidural space of cadavers reveal only minimal lateral spread, even with very large volumes (60-80 ml). Such lateral spread as there is, is confined to the cuffs surrounding the spinal nerves and does not appear to reach the paravertebral space (Fig. 1:25a and b).

Fig. 1:25 a. and b. Antero-posterior radiograph following the epidural injection of 80 ml of radio-opaque fluid in a cadaver. Note limited lateral spread confined to the nerve cuffs.

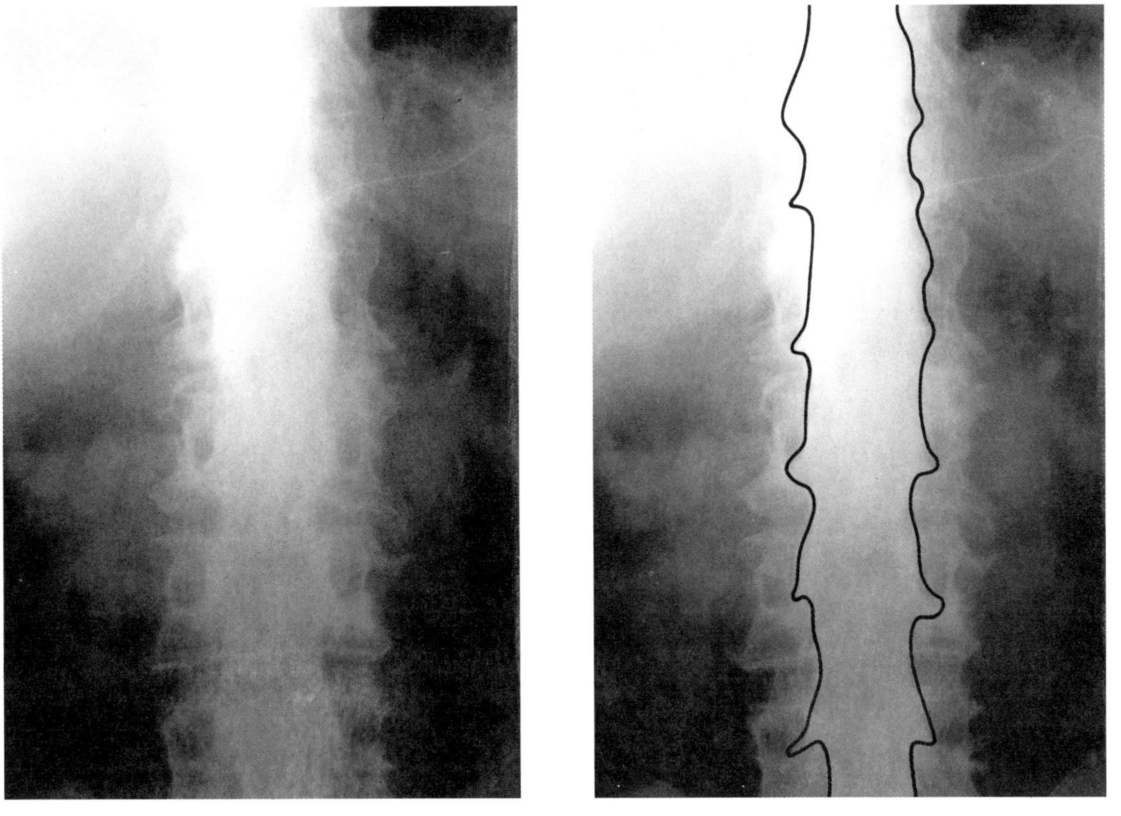

Autonomic nervous system

Epidural anaesthesia can cause a widespread blockade of both sympathetic and parasympathetic nerves. This has considerable effects, mainly on the control of the circulation but also on the normal function of the gastrointestinal tract. In addition, afferent autonomic nerves are involved in the appreciation of painful stimuli in the abdomen and must be blocked if total analgesia is to be achieved.

Finally, blockade of the autonomic supply to endocrine glands can greatly modify the response of these glands to surgical stress.

Sympathetic nervous system

Efferent impulses from the central nervous system to the blood vessels and organs supplied by sympathetic nerves must travel along both preganglionic and postganglionic nerves. Thus two nerve fibres are involved with a connecting synapse within a ganglion. The ganglia are located in the sympathetic chain and in the large plexuses within the thorax and abdomen, such as the cardiac, coeliac and hypogastric plexuses (Fig. 1:26).

Preganglionic nerves arise from nerve cells in the lateral column of the grey matter of the spinal cord. They leave the spinal cord through the spinal nerves from T_1 to L_2. Some authorities claim that they may also arise in the cervical spinal nerves. Just lateral to the intervertebral foramina, the preganglionic nerve fibres, which are lightly myelinated, leave the spinal nerve to become the white rami communicantes which run to the sympathetic chain. Within the chain they may go up or down to reach a synapse within the appropriate ganglia. Many do not synapse in the chain but leave it to reach ganglia in the large plexuses.

The sympathetic chain runs the length of the spinal column along the anterolateral aspect of the vertebral bodies. In the cervical region the collections of ganglia make up the superior cervical, the middle cervical and the stellate ganglia. In the thorax the sympathetic chain gives rise to the splanchnic nerves (greater, lesser and lowest), which penetrate the diaphragm to reach the coeliac plexus. In the abdomen there are connections with the coeliac, aortic and hypogastric plexuses. The chain ends in the pelvis on the anterior surface of the sacrum. The unmyelinated postganglionic nerves arising from the ganglia are widely distributed to all the organs receiving a sympathetic nerve supply. Many run back to the spinal nerves via the grey rami communicantes and reach structures within the distribution of the spinal nerves. These nerves supply the blood vessels as well as organs within the skin, such as the sweat glands. It will be seen that while only 14 spinal nerves (T_1-L_2) give rise to preganglionic nerves, all spinal nerves receive postganglionic fibres. Postganglionic nerves from the stellate ganglia are distributed to the head along the major blood vessels.

The heart, lungs and viscera receive their postganglionic fibres more directly through branches which leave the large plexuses.

Fig. 1:26 Schematic diagram of the efferent component of the sympathetic nervous system.

1. Superior cervical ganglion
2. Middle cervical ganglion
3. Stellate ganglion
4. Coeliac ganglion
5. Superior mesenteric ganglion
6. Inferior mesenteric ganglion
7. Superior hypogastric plexus

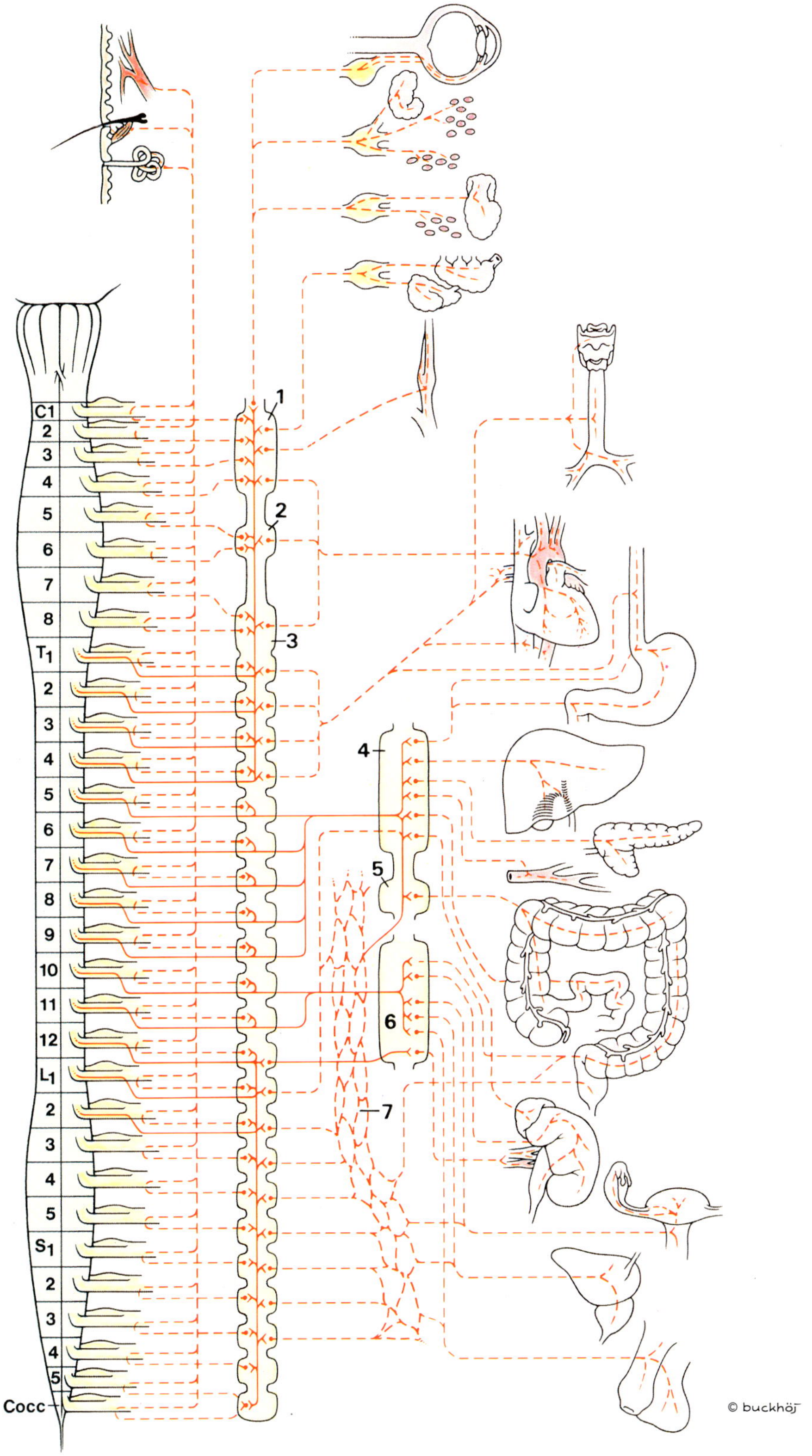
C1
2
3
4
5
6
7
8
T1
2
3
4
5
6
7
8
9
10
11
12
L1
2
3
4
5
S1
2
3
4
5
Cocc
1
2
3
4
5
6
7
© buckhöj

The segmental distribution of the sympathetic nerves is as follows:

Head, neck and upper limbs	T_{1-5}
Heart	T_{1-5}
Lungs	T_{2-4}
Oesophagus	T_{5-6}
Stomach	T_{6-10}
Small intestine	T_{9-10}
Large bowel	T_{11}-L_2
Liver and gall bladder	T_{7-9}
Pancreas and spleen	T_{6-10}
Kidney and ureter	T_{10}-L_2
Adrenal glands	T_8-L_1
Testis and ovary	T_{10-11}
Bladder	T_{11}-L_2
Prostate	T_{11}-L_1
Uterus	T_{10}-L_1

Parasympathetic nervous system

Efferent nerves of the parasympathetic system run either in cranial nerves or in the 2nd, 3rd and 4th sacral nerves (Fig. 1:27). The vagus nerve is the most important cranial nerve carrying parasympathetic efferent nerves, but these also exist in the oculomotor, the facial, the glossopharyngeal and the accessory nerves. Preganglionic fibres run all the way to the various organs they supply. Synapses occur in the walls of these organs with very short postganglionic fibres.

The vagus nerve supplies the heart, lungs, oesophagus and gastrointestinal tract down to the transverse colon. The sacral parasympathetic nerves are distributed with the corresponding sympathetic nerves to the large bowel below the transverse colon, the bladder, the sphincters and the reproductive organs.

Unlike all other autonomic nerves, the cranial parasympathetic nerves, and especially the vagus nerve, cannot be affected by epidural blockade.

Fig. 1:27 Schematic diagram of the efferent component of the parasympathetic nervous system.

1. Pharyngeal plexus
2. Superior vagal ganglion
3. Inferior vagal ganglion
4. Coeliac ganglion
5. Coeliac plexus
6. Mesenteric ganglion
7. Superior hypogastric plexus
8. Inferior hypogastric plexus

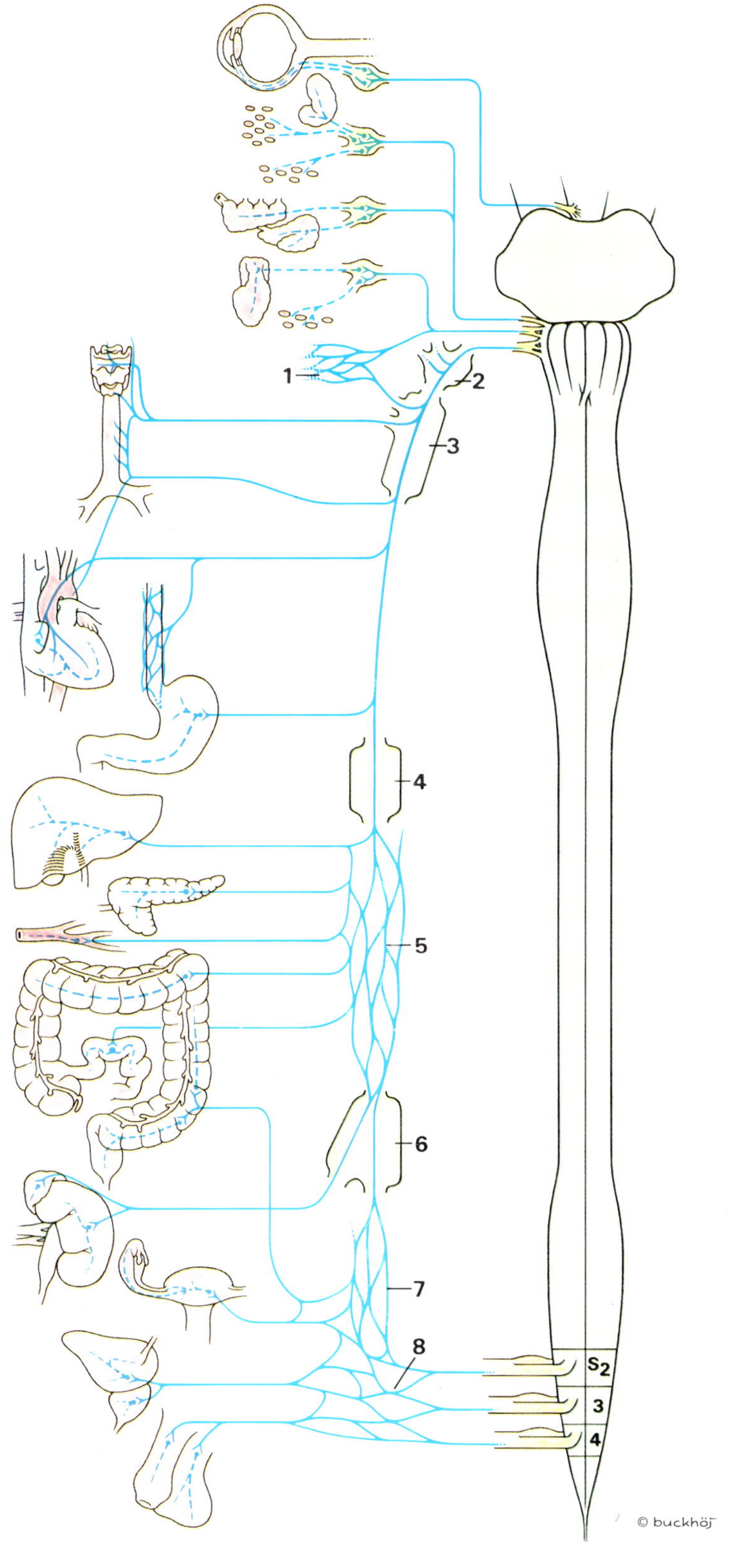
1
2
3
4
5
6
7
8
S2
3
4
© buckhöj

Autonomic afferent nerves

Distributed with the efferent nerves of both the sympathetic and parasympathetic systems are afferent fibres whose nerve cells are located in the dorsal root ganglia (Fig. 1:28a and b). These fibres are responsible for the afferent arcs of visceral reflexes. They are concerned with sensations such as hunger, nausea, bladder distension and uterine contractions. Certain kinds of pain are mediated through these nerves, such as colic and labour pain. They are usually activated by excessive stretching or contraction of unstriated muscle but may also respond to inflammation (e.g. peritonitis) or ischaemia (e.g. angina).

Fig. 1:28b. Afferent parasympathetic nerve pathways from the stomach via the vagus nerve.

1. Superior cervical ganglion
2. Middle cervical ganglion
3. Stellate ganglion
4. Superior vagal ganglion
5. Inferior vagal ganglion

Fig. 1:28a. Schematic diagram of afferent sympathetic pathways from heart.

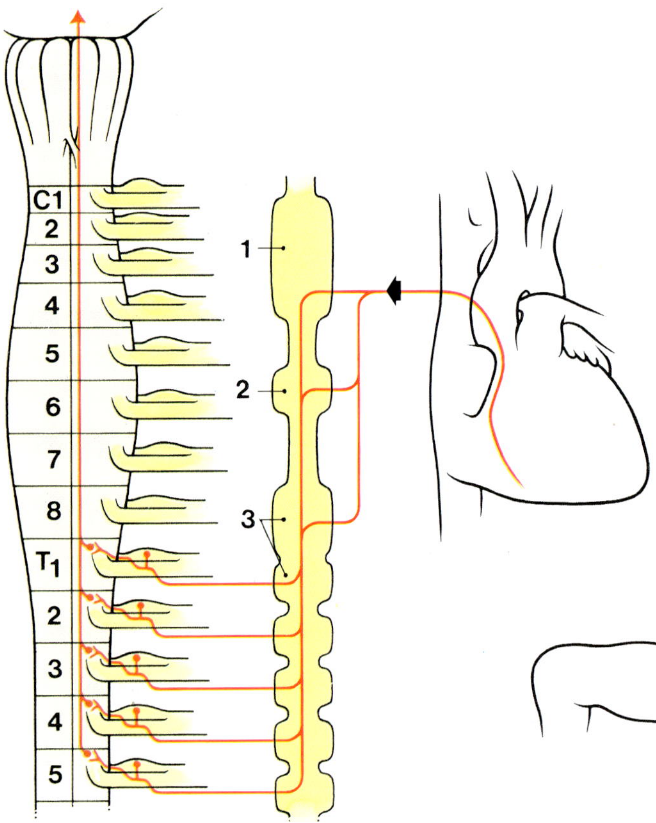

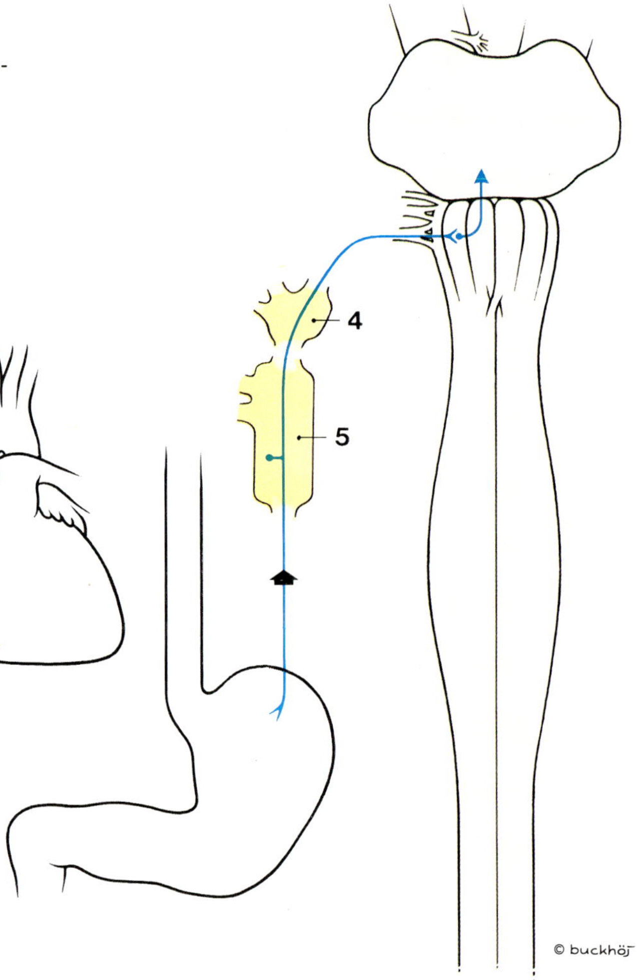

Chapter 1

References & Bibliography

Nieuwenhuys, R., Voogd, J., van Huijzen, C. (1979). The Human Central Nervous System., Springer-Verlag, Heidelberg.

Petren, T. (1958). Lärobok i Anatomi, Fack och Specialböcker, Stockholm.

Sobotta, J., Becher, H. (1962). Atlas der Anatomie des Menschen., Urban & Schwartzenberg., München-Berlin.

Warwick, R., Williams, P.L. (1980). Gray's Anatomy. Churchill Livingstone, Edinburgh.

2. Physiological considerations

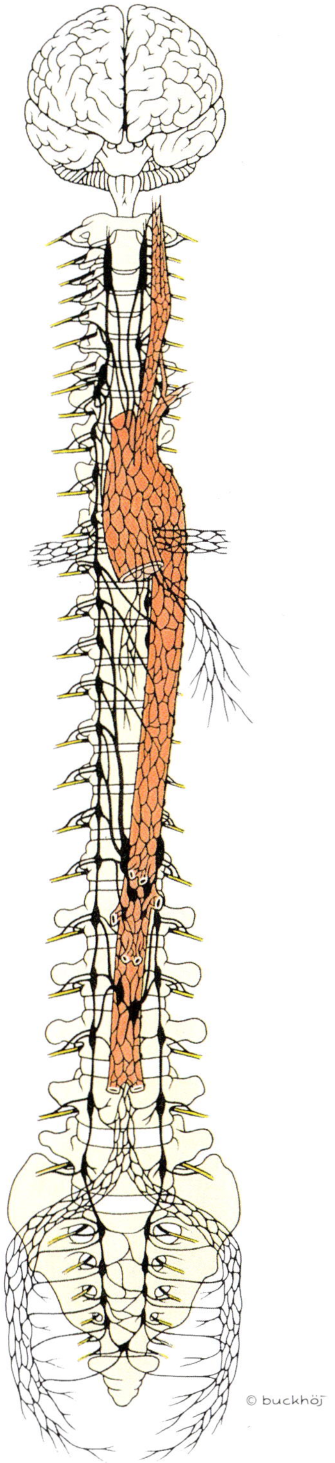

Mechanism of epidural anaesthesia

The possible sites of action of local anaesthetic drugs administered into the epidural space include the spinal nerve trunks in the paravertebral space, the dorsal root ganglia, the dorsal and ventral spinal roots and the spinal cord itself.

Mixed spinal nerves in the paravertebral space

It was originally believed that the dura mater was impermeable to local anaesthetic solutions and that epidural anaesthesia was essentially analogous to multiple spinal nerve blocks. The mixed spinal nerves which traverse the epidural space originate from the union of the dorsal and ventral spinal roots. They leave the epidural space by way of the intervertebral foramina (Fig. 2:1). Early investigators believed that local anaesthetic solutions injected into the epidural space escaped through the intervertebral foramina and caused conduction blockade in the mixed nerves in the paravertebral spaces. Support for this hypothesis was obtained from studies in which radio-opaque material injected into the epidural space was interpreted as escaping from the epidural space through the intervertebral foramina. More recent studies (see p. 27) reveal very little lateral spread, indicating that the epidural space is essentially a closed space.

It was thought that greater volumes of anaesthetic solutions were required to achieve the same segmental level of epidural blockade in young patients as in older patients. This was believed to be related to the fact that in young patients local anaesthetic could escape easily into the paravertebral space. However, with better controlled studies, the relationship between the spread of anaesthesia and the volume of

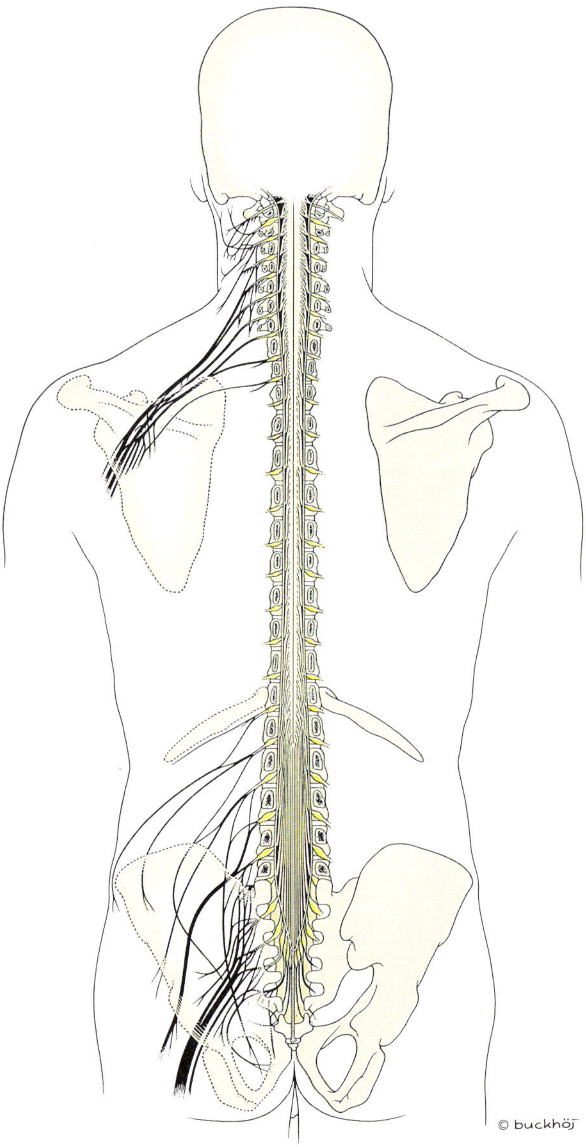

Fig. 2:1 Entire length of vertebral column showing the spinal cord, spinal roots and mixed spinal nerves which exit through the intervertebral foramina. All of these nerve structures represent possible sites of action of epidurally administered local anaesthetics.

solution injected into the epidural space of young and old patients is not well correlated. Currently it is believed that multiple mixed spinal nerve blocks in the paravertebral space probably play a minor role in the mechanism of epidural anaesthesia.

Dorsal root ganglion

The dorsal root ganglia would appear to be a logical site for the action of local anaesthetic agents injected into the epidural space (Fig. 2:2). They are located in the dural root sleeves which pass directly through the epidural space. Thus, local anaesthetics could easily diffuse from the epidural space to the ganglia and inhibit excitation of ganglion cells.

Fig. 2:2 Cross-section of the spinal cord and spinal roots and the location of the dorsal root ganglion. The ganglion is variable in position and can be more lateral than is shown in the figure.

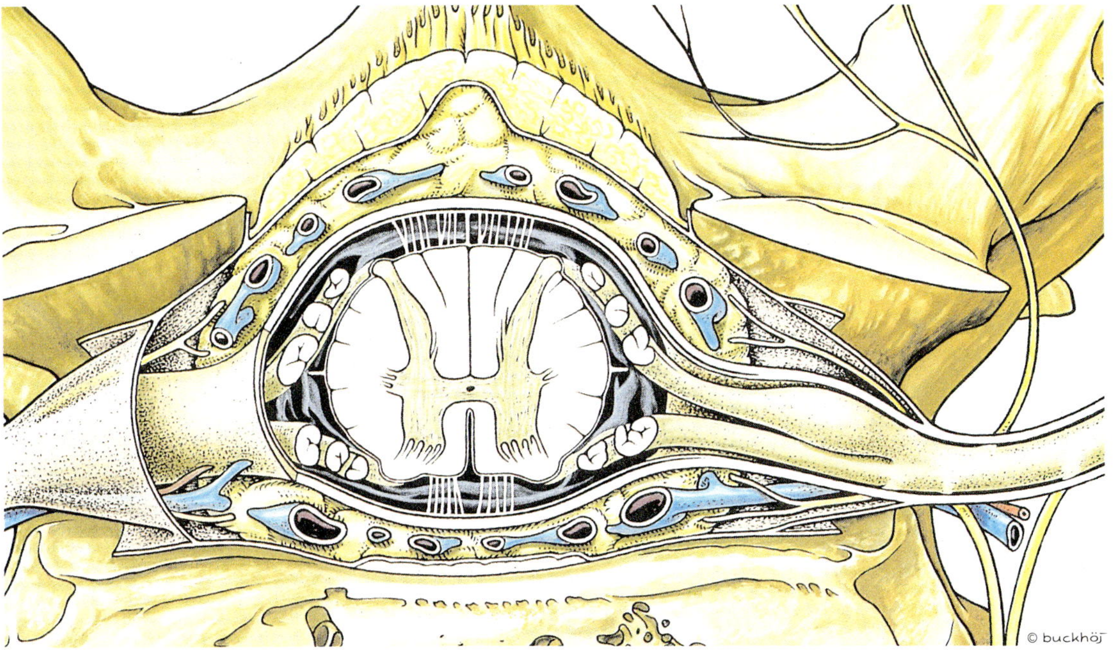

However, tissue distribution studies of radioactive lidocaine administered into the subarachnoid space have shown that minimal concentrations of lidocaine are present in the dorsal ganglia compared with other subdural neural structures (Fig. 2:3). This suggests that dorsal root ganglion inhibition is not a primary determinant of epidural anaesthesia. Moreover, local anaesthetics are known to cause inhibition of sodium conductance and a decrease in the rate and degree of depolarisation in axonal membranes while exerting minimal effects on ganglion cells. Thus, it appears unlikely that the dorsal root ganglia are primarily involved in the mechanism of epidural anaesthesia.

Fig. 2:3 Cross-section of spinal cord, spinal roots and dorsal root ganglia showing concentration of local anaesthetics in each structure following epidural administration. (Modified from Bromage)

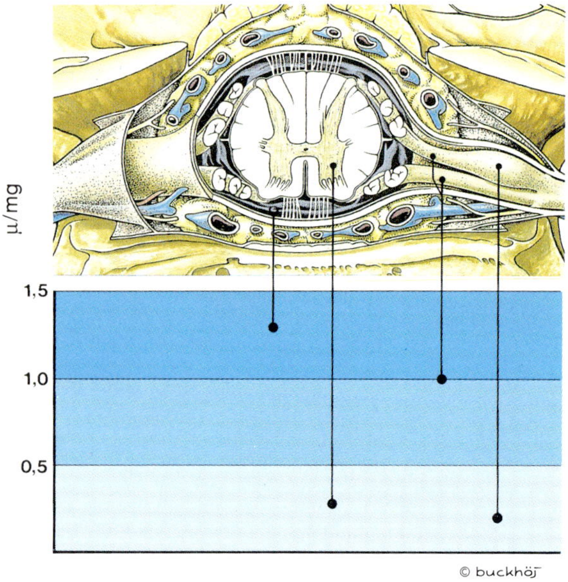

Spinal roots

The dorsal and the ventral spinal roots are ideally located vis-à-vis the epidural space and would appear to be particularly susceptible to the action of epidurally administered local anaesthetic agents owing to the unique anatomy of the membranous structures around the spinal roots where they join to form the spinal nerve (Fig. 2:2). In this area the dura mater is relatively thin and some believe that arachnoid granulations are present which increase the surface area available for diffusion of anaesthetic agents from the epidural space into the subarachnoid space. As has been discussed on p. 20, arachnoid granulations are only present in relatively few dural cuffs in man. Nevertheless, local anaesthetic agents administered into the epidural space could easily cross the thin dura around the spinal roots. The concentration of local anaesthetic agent in the vicinity of the spinal roots would soon exceed the minimum effective anaesthetic level required for conduction blockade. Indeed, it has been shown that local anaesthetics administered intrathecally are concentrated to a greater extent in spinal roots than either dorsal root ganglion or the spinal cord itself. Furthermore, local anaesthetic agents administered into the epidural space have been found in spinal roots to an even greater extent than was observed following the subarachnoid injection of these agents (Fig. 2:3). Additional evidence favouring the spinal roots as the initial site of action of epidurally administered local anaesthetics is obtained from clinical studies evaluating the onset pattern of epidural blockade. A significant delay in onset of anaesthesia at the S_1 and S_2 dermatomal levels is almost invariably observed following the epidural administration of various local anaesthetics (Fig. 2:4a). In some cases, little or no anaesthesia is present at the S_1 and S_2 level, although adequate anaesthesia is obtained above and below those dermatomes (Fig. 2:4b). This

Fig. 2:4 Distribution of epidural analgesia with time in two patients given etidocaine with epinephrine. a. Shows lack of analgesia at the S_1-S_2 spinal segments. b. Shows delay in onset and early regression of analgesia at the S_1-S_2 spinal segments.

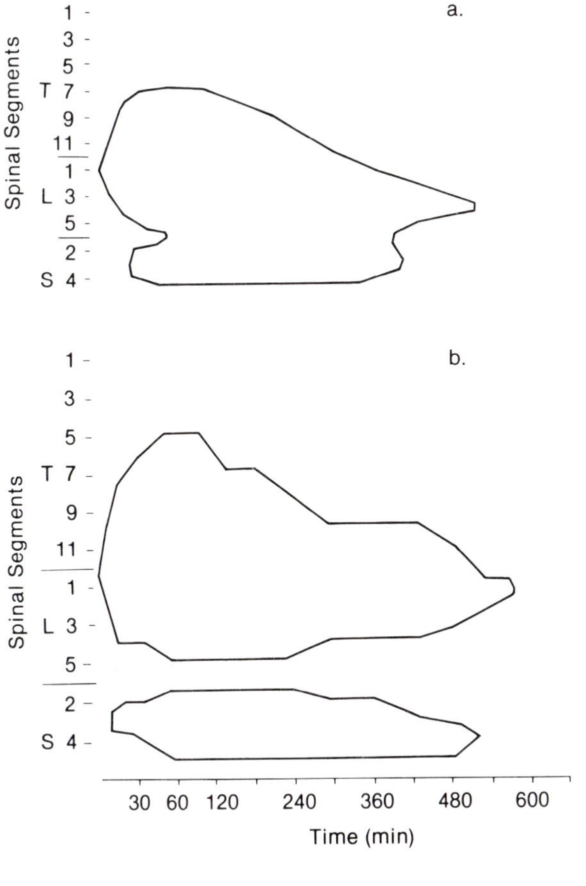

delay or failure to achieve anaesthesia in the S_1-S_2 region is correlated with the size of the nerve roots in that area. For example, in one study the diameter of spinal nerve roots was shown to increase from 2.2 mm at the T_{12} level to a maximum of 3.8 mm at S_1 and subsequently decrease to a diameter of 1.0 mm at the S_5 level (Fig. 2:5). The increased fibre size of the nerve roots is believed to be related to a greater density of connective tissue. As a result the rate of diffusion of local anaesthetic agents to the nerve membrane receptor sites is decreased in these large nerve roots. The favourable anatomical location of the spinal roots, the anatomy of the arachnoid membrane in this region, the significant uptake of local anaesthetics by spinal roots and the correlation between the onset of epidural anaesthesia and the thickness of spinal roots strongly suggest that the spinal roots are involved to a great extent in the mechanism of epidural anaesthesia.

Fig. 2:5 Diagram depicts difference in cross-sectional diameter of spinal roots from the T_{12} to the S_5 spinal segment.

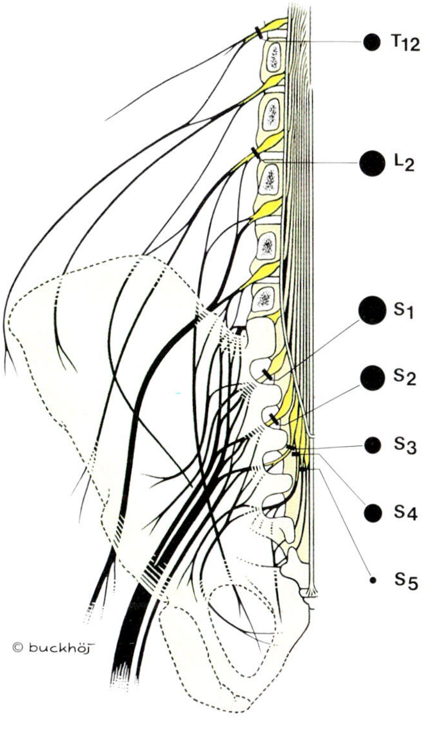

Spinal cord

For many years the spinal cord was ignored as a possible site of action for anaesthetic drugs administered into the epidural space. The dura mater, which separates the subdural and the epidural spaces, consists of relatively thick, fibrous tissue which was believed to be impermeable to the movement of drugs from one space to the other (Fig. 1:17, p. 19). However, a number of studies in animals and man clearly indicate that the dura mater does not represent a barrier to the movement of various substances between the epidural and the subarachnoid spaces. Investigations with procaine and radioactive lidocaine demonstrated that local anaesthetic agents injected into the epidural space rapidly reach the cerebrospinal fluid. Subsequently, tissue distribution studies following both intrathecal and epidural administration of labelled local anaesthetics have shown that these agents can penetrate the spinal cord. However, the concentration of local anaesthetics in the spinal cord following either intrathecal or epidural administration was less than that found in the spinal roots (Fig. 2:3). Autoradiographic studies in dogs indicate that epidurally administered lidocaine diffuses through the dura mater into the cerebrospinal fluid and penetrates into peripheral areas of the spinal cord.

The depth of penetration of local anaesthetic drugs into the spinal cord appears to be related to the physicochemical properties of the agent employed. A highly lipid soluble drug such as etidocaine has been found to reach a greater depth in the spinal cord than less lipid soluble local anaesthetic agents.

In spite of diffusion into the spinal cord, the cord is not believed to be the initial site of action of local anaesthetics following epidural administration since the dermatomal onset patterns of epidural anaesthesia differ from that observed following subarachnoid blockade. Subarachnoid administration of local anaesthetic agents is not associated with delay or absence of anaesthesia in sacral segments as is frequently observed following injection of anaesthetic solution into the lumbar epidural space. On the other hand, during the recovery phase from epidural blockade, analgesia regresses from the higher to the lower dermatomes in a caudad direction, similar to the regression observed following subarachnoid blockade. This suggests that spinal cord blockade does occur following epidural administration of local anaesthetic agents, but the initial onset of anaesthesia is probably related to inhibition of conduction in spinal roots.

In summary, the spread and diffusion of local anaesthetic agents administered into the epidural space and subsequently the mechanism of epidural anaesthesia is relatively complex in nature (Fig. 2:6). Most of the initial spread of epidurally administered local anaesthetic solutions involves diffusion through the relatively thin dura and arachnoid membranes in the region of the spinal roots near the junction where they form the spinal nerve. This results in a high concentration of local anaesthetics surrounding the spinal roots such that the initial segmental onset of epidural anaesthesia is probably related to conduction block of the spinal roots in the dural sleeves. Subsequently, diffusion of local anaesthetics from the epidural space through the dura mater into the cerebrospinal fluid occurs. Local anaesthetic agents reaching the cerebrospinal fluid penetrate the periphery of the spinal cord and thus contribute to the degree of nerve blockade. The depth and duration of epidural blockade is related in part to the amount of drug taken up by the spinal roots and the spinal cord, which is a function of the total concentration of the drug administered. The degree of sensory and motor blockade is also a function of the physicochemical properties of the specific agent employed. In particular, the more lipid soluble agents such as etidocaine will probably inhibit conduction in the large myelinated A-alpha motor fibres in the dorsal roots to a greater extent than will less lipid soluble local anaesthetics. Furthermore, the depth of penetration into the spinal cord is also influenced by the lipid solubility of the various agents which, in turn, will determine the relative degree of sensory analgesia and motor blockade since sensory fibres are believed to be located more towards the periphery while motor tracts are located deeper within the spinal cord.

Fig. 2:6 A summary of the possible diffusion pathways of epidurally administered local anaesthetic agents to various neural structures.

1. Through dura to CSF
2. CSF to cord
3. Dural root sleeves to nerve roots and cord
4. Dural root sleeves to spinal nerve

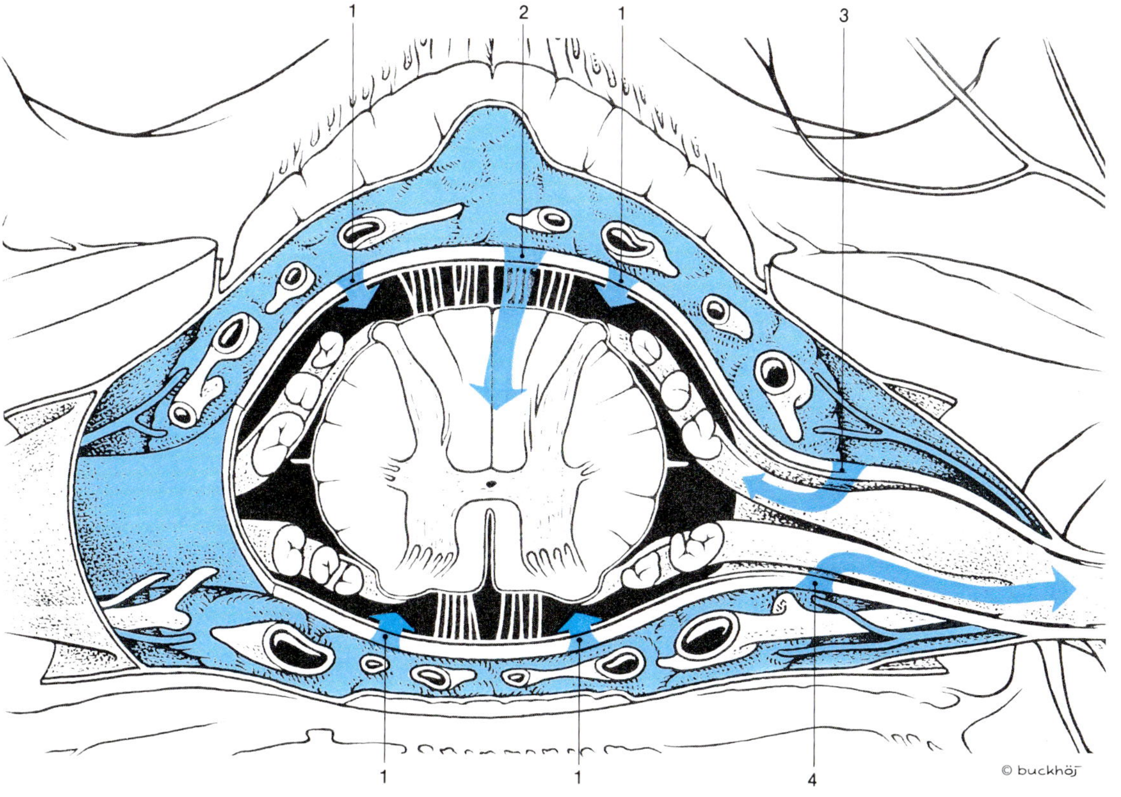

Sensory afferent pathways

A primary aim of epidural anaesthesia is to prevent the conduction of nociceptive impulses from the surgical or obstetrical site to the brain. A variety of specialised receptors or bare nerve endings exist in the skin and other tissues, including the viscera. These receptors and nerve endings respond to noxious stimuli as well as mechanical, thermal and chemical stimulation. Following the activation of these specialised receptors or bare nerve endings, impulses are conducted along specific fibre types within peripheral nerves. Three specific fibre types (A, B and C) have been identified, based primarily on their diameter and the rate of impulse conduction (Fig. 2:7).

The A fibres are the largest and most rapidly conducting, and have been subdivided into various subgroups. The A-alpha and A-beta fibres are approximately 5-20 µm in diameter and conduct impulses at a rate of 40-120 $m.sec^{-1}$. These fibres are heavily myelinated, respond to mechanical stimuli primarily, and are located in skin, joints, muscles and viscera. The A-gamma fibres are 4-8 µm in diameter, conduct impulses at 15-40 $m.sec^{-1}$, and respond to touch. The A-delta fibres are the smallest of the myelinated fibres in the A group. They vary in size from 1 to 5 µm, conduct impulses at a rate of 5-15 $m.sec^{-1}$ and originate in the skin, joints, viscera and blood vessel walls. Approximately 75% of the A-delta fibres respond to mechanical and thermal stimulation, while 25% are nociceptive and activated by noxious stimuli.

The B fibres are lightly myelinated nerves with a diameter of 1-3 µm. They are capable of conducting impulses at a rate of 3-14 $m.sec^{-1}$. The B fibres are located in the preganglionic portion of the autonomic nervous system and are involved in the conduction of both sympathetic and parasympathetic impulses.

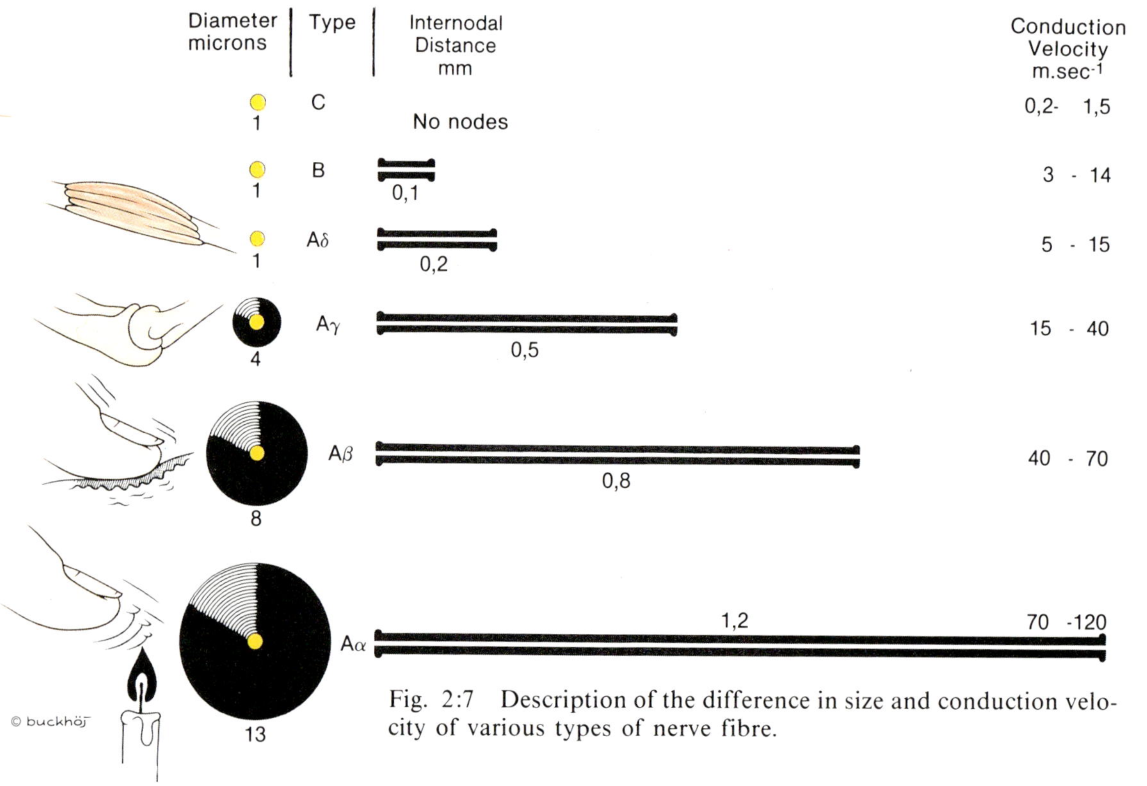

Fig. 2:7 Description of the difference in size and conduction velocity of various types of nerve fibre.

The C fibres represent the smallest fibres of the peripheral nervous system. They are unmyelinated with a diameter size of 0.5-1 μm. They conduct impulses at a rate of 0.2-1.5 m. sec^{-1}. Approximately 50% of the C fibres respond to mechanical and thermal stimulation, while the remaining 50% are nociceptive in nature. Thus, both A-delta fibres and C fibres transmit nociceptive impulses. Sharp, intense pain is transmitted primarily by way of the A-delta fibres, while dull pain sensations are transmitted via the smaller C fibres.

The nociceptive impulses which are conducted along A-delta and C fibres reach the spinal cord by way of the dorsal spinal roots. From here they enter the region of the dorsal horn (Fig. 8: a and b). Some of the sensory fibres pass directly through the dorsal horn and cross to the contralateral spinothalamic tract. Other sensory fibres form synaptic connections within the dorsal horn. The dorsal horn has been divided anatomically into various laminae. Sensory fibres of the A-delta and C types from skin and viscera terminate at synaptic junctions in laminae I and V and probably also laminae IV and VI. Fibres which terminate in lamina I activate multiple neuronal paths which pass through laminae II and III and ultimately impinge on the neuronal structures in lamina V. Other sensory fibres pass directly to lamina V and impinge on the same neuronal bodies. Postganglionic fibres from lamina V then pass to the ipsilateral and contralateral spinothalamic tracts.

The dorsal horn is a complex area of neuronal connections where the integration and modulation of noxious impulses occur, primarily in laminae II and III, which constitute the substantia gelatinosa. Noxious impulses conducted along A-delta and C fibres arrive at the substantia gelatinosa by way of synaptic connections from lamina I, where most of the peripheral sensory fibres terminate. These noxious impulses would proceed uninterrupted to the ipsilateral and contralateral spinothalamic tracts if it were

Fig. 2:8a. Depicts sensory afferent fibres entering the dorsal horn of the spinal column. Synaptic connections occur in the dorsal horn following which post-synaptic fibres leave the dorsal horn and travel by various pathways to the brain. b. Shows a detailed diagram of the dorsal horn with the various laminae where the numerous synaptic connections occur.

1. Dorsal column
2. Dorsal root
3. Dorsal root ganglion
4. Ventral spinothalamic fasciculi
5. Substantia gelatinosa
6. Large cutaneous fibres
7. Small cutaneous fibres
8. Visceral fibres
9. To contralateral spinothalamic tract
10. To ipsilateral spinothalamic tract

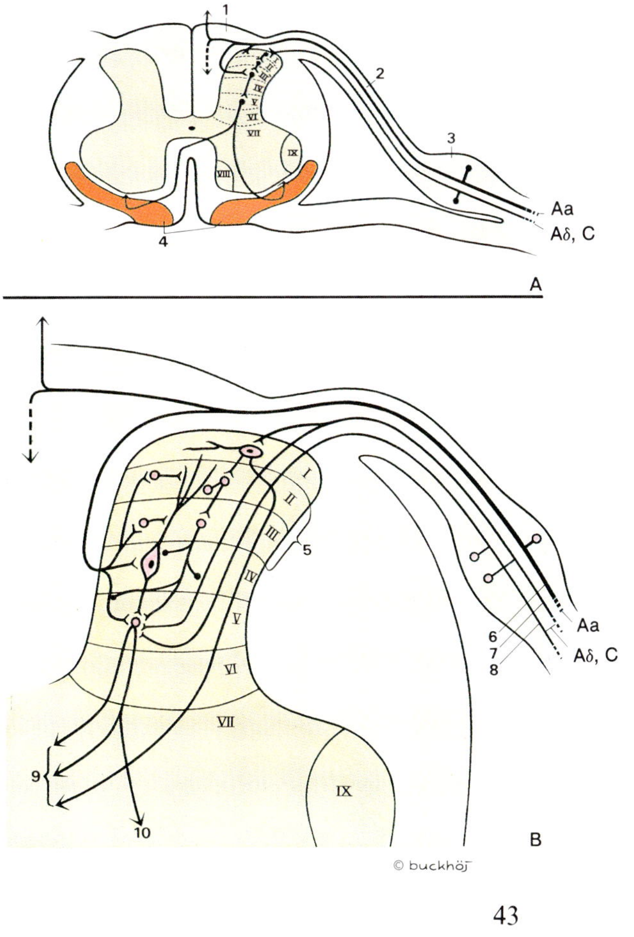

Fig. 2:9 Diagram showing the pathways followed by the lateral spinothalamic tract from the spinal cord to the brain.

1. Limbic forebrain structure
2. Thalamus
3. Hypothalamus
4. Reticular formation

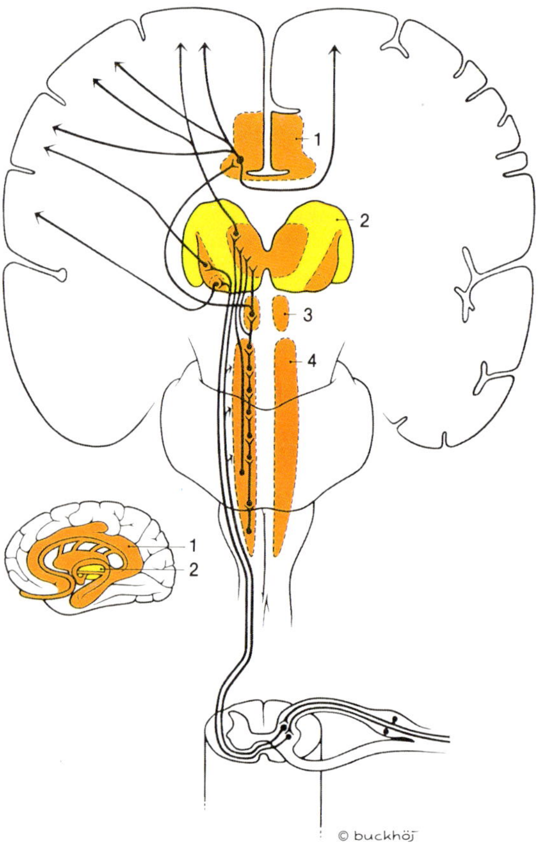

not for the modulating effect of impulses from large A-alpha fibres. These large myelinated fibres from the dorsal spinal roots enter the dorsal columns and divide into ascending and descending tracts (Fig. 2:8). In addition, a branch of these large fibres penetrates the dorsal horn at lamina IV and subdivides into small fibres which impinge on neurons in laminae II and III, the substantia gelatinosa, and also to a lesser extent laminae I and V. These large fibres are believed to be responsible for the inhibition of postsynaptic neurons in laminae II and III and thus modify the number of noxious impulses which pass through this area to the spinothalamic tracts and then to the cerebral cortex, where pain perception occurs.

This interaction of large and small fibres in the substantia gelatinosa is the basic element in the gate control theory proposed by Melzack and Wall. Some of the large fibres are excitatory in nature and allow impulses to proceed through the synaptic areas in laminae II and III as though a gate were open. Other large fibres are inhibitory in nature and their action is analogous to the closing of a gate which diminishes the number of noxious impulses that can be transmitted.

The lateral spinothalamic tract (Fig. 2:9) is the primary afferent pathway for sensory impulses and can be divided into the neospinothalamic and paleospinothalamic tracts. The neospinothalamic tract proceeds directly to the posterior thalamus where it synapses with neurons that pass to the cerebral cortex (Fig. 2:10). The paleospinothalamic tract sends numerous branches which synapse with intermediary neurons in the reticular formation. From there these intermediary neurons pass to the hypothalamus, where they synapse again with neurons which proceed to the thalamus and from there to the cerebral cortex (Fig. 2:11). Although the spinothalamic tract is the primary afferent pathway for noxious impulses, nociceptive impulses can also reach the cerebral cortex by other ascending afferent systems, such as the medial lemniscus and the reticular spinal tract, while other multisynaptic afferent tracts transmit impulses to the cortex via the reticular formation and thalamus.

Fig. 2:10 Diagram showing the pathway followed by the neospinothalamic tract from the spinal cord to the brain.

1. Thalamus

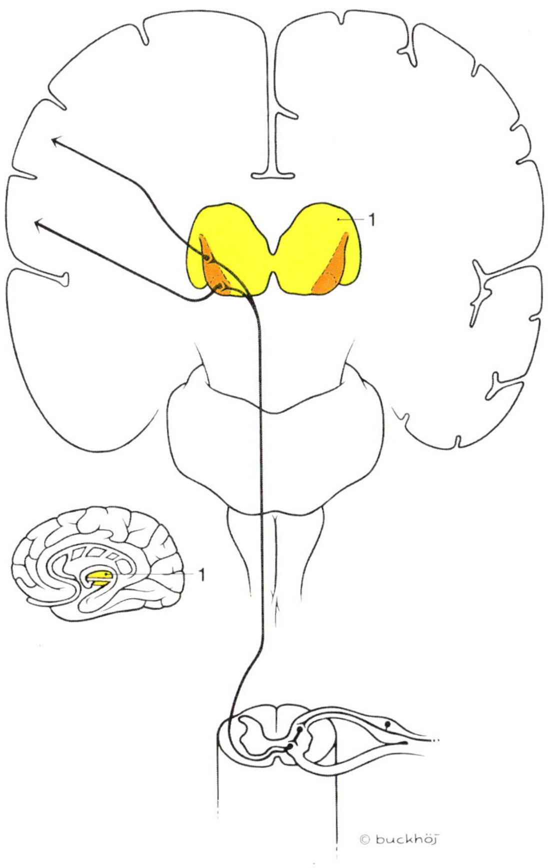

Fig. 2:11 Diagram showing the pathway followed by the paleospinothalamic tract from the spinal cord to the brain.

1. Limbic forebrain structure
2. Thalamus
3. Hypothalamus
4. Reticular formation

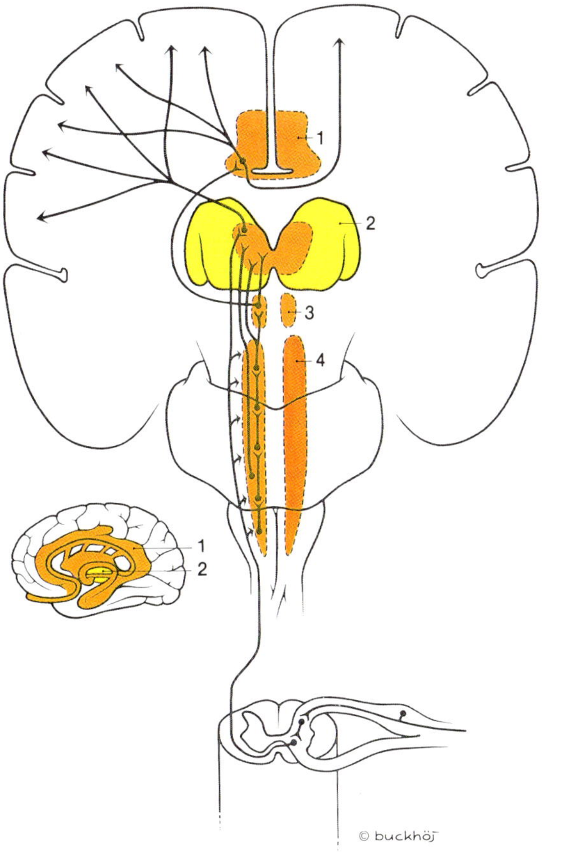

Descending pathways

Descending pathways from the cerebral cortex serve several functions. These pathways in the corticospinal tract and reticulospinal tract may enter the dorsal horn at all levels of the spinal cord (Fig. 2:12). These fibres are believed to be both inhibitory and excitatory in nature. They impinge on synaptic structures in the substantia gelatinosa and thereby modulate the passage of nociceptive impulses. Other fibres may proceed from the cortex and descend directly by way of the corticospinal tract or via the thalamus, the reticular formation and the reticulospinal tract to the spinal cord and leave through the ventral horns and the ventral spinal roots to reach the structures which they innervate.

Fibres of the autonomic nervous system also descend from the cortex to the spinal cord and leave by way of the ventral roots. The autonomic pathways are described in detail on p. 28.

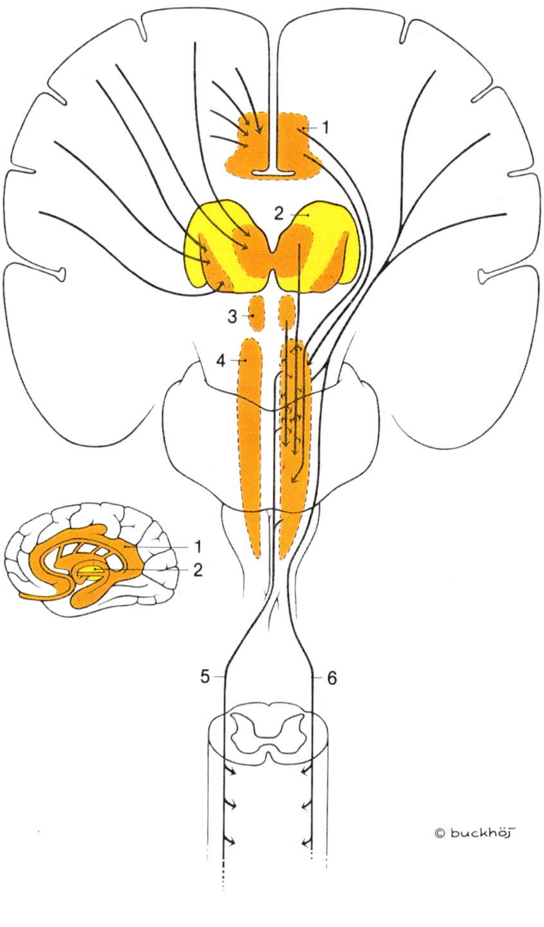

Fig. 2:12 Diagram showing descending pathways from the cerebral cortex to the spinal cord.

1. Limbic forebrain structure
2. Thalamus
3. Hypothalamus
4. Reticular formation
5. Reticulospinal tract
6. Corticulospinal tract

Physiological effects of epidural blockade

Administration of local anaesthetics in sufficient dosage into the epidural space will interrupt the passage of sensory, motor and autonomic impulses in both dorsal and ventral spinal roots, and to some extent in the cord itself. The sensitivity of various nerve fibres to local anaesthetics is related to the size and type of the nerve fibre, the quantity of local anaesthetic administered epidurally and the physicochemical properties of the local anaesthetic agent. Recent in vitro studies in isolated nerves have suggested that the classical concept relating local anaesthetic blockade to fibre size may be incorrect. These studies have shown that large myelinated fibres are more sensitive to local anaesthetic blockade than smaller, unmyelinated fibres. However, in vivo diffusion of local anaesthetics to the membrane receptor site and interaction with those receptors are both involved in determining the apparent sensitivity of various nerve fibres to local anaesthetic blockade. Thus, the small, unmyelinated fibres are usually affected initially following epidural injection owing to the lack of diffusion barriers. The larger, heavily myelinated motor fibres of the A type are usually more resistant to block owing to the thick myelin sheath surrounding them, which serves as a barrier to the diffusion of local anaesthetics.

As will be discussed in a later chapter, certain drugs which possess a relatively low pKa and are very lipid soluble, such as etidocaine, will penetrate motor fibres readily. Thus, little difference in the sensitivity of A-alpha, A-delta and C fibres to etidocaine is seen following epidural administration of this agent. The rate of blockade of preganglionic autonomic B fibres also varies according to the dosage of local anaesthetic and the specific agent administered into the epidural space. Sympathetic block sufficient to cause systemic hypotension rarely occurs before sensory anaesthesia is well established. Thus, sensory analgesia is usually the first indication of successful epidural blockade.

Haemodynamic effects

Interruption of sympathetic impulses can lead to cardiovascular alterations following the establishment of epidural anaesthesia (Fig. 2:13). In most patients, despite autonomic blockade, cardiovascular changes are not very marked. On the other hand, profound hypotension may be observed in some patients following the onset of epidural anaesthesia. The changes in blood pressure, heart rate and cardiac output are related to the level of blockade, the amount of drug administered, the specific local anaesthetic agent employed, the inclusion of a vasoconstrictor in the anaesthetic solution and the cardiovascular status of the patient.

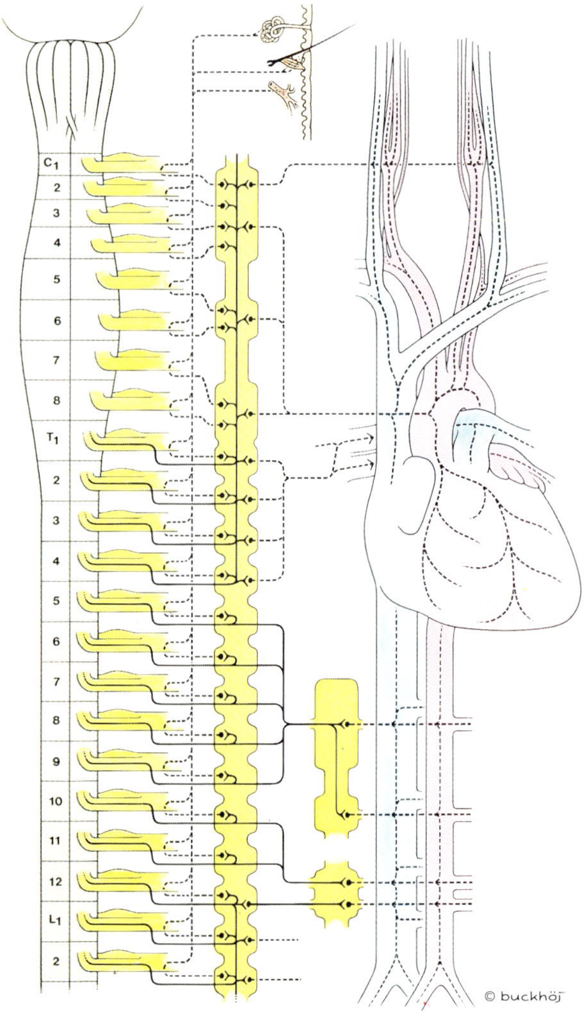

Fig. 2:13 Diagram showing the efferent innervation of the heart and blood vessels by the sympathetic nervous system.

Level of block

The higher the block, the greater the number of sympathetic fibres that are affected, leading to a reduction in vascular tone. Thus peripheral resistance decreases, but a fall in arterial pressure may be prevented by vasoconstriction in unblocked segments. Thus, blocks below T_5 are seldom associated with marked hypotension (Fig. 2:14a). Higher blocks, however, will not only prevent compensatory vasoconstriction but also affect the cardiac sympathetic nerves which arise in the T_{1-5} segments. At these dermatomal levels of block, a fall in heart rate and cardiac output may occur (Fig. 2:14c). The blockade of sympathetic fibres to the heart and the failure to block the vagus nerves can cause vasovagal attacks which are associated with profound bradycardia and, in some patients, with transient cardiac arrest. This may, in fact, represent the most common cause of profound hypotension following high levels of epidural anaesthesia. As the veins forming the capacitance vessels will also be affected by the sympathetic block, venous pooling can occur if the venous return is obstructed by gravity or abdominal tumours or by the pregnant uterus. Thus, patients are very susceptible to the head-up posture, which causes expansion of the capacitance vessels and can lead to a marked decrease in venous return and cardiac output (Fig. 2:14b).

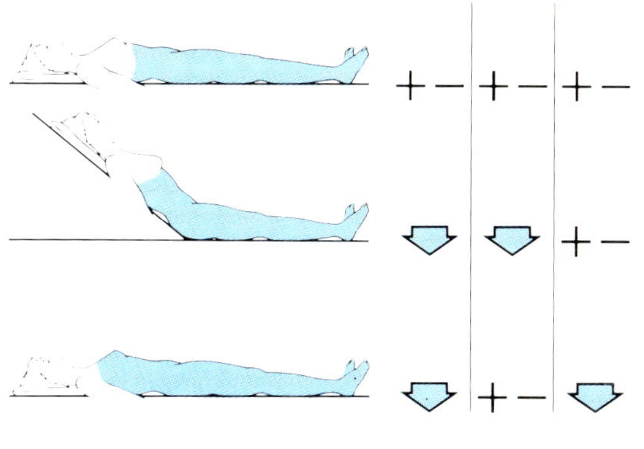

Fig. 2:14 Diagram showing relationship between level of block, patient position, and changes in various cardiovascular variables.

a. Block to T_5 horizontal
b. Block to T_5 head up
c. Block to T_5 horizontal

Drug dosage

Relatively large amounts of local anaesthetic drug are required to achieve a satisfactory degree of epidural blockade. The local anaesthetic agents are absorbed rather rapidly and may produce systemic effects involving the cardiovascular system. Most local anaesthetic agents produce a biphasic effect on the cardiovascular system. For example, it has been shown that blood levels of lidocaine of up to 4 $\mu g.ml^{-1}$ following epidural blockade resulted in a slight increase in blood pressure owing mainly to an increase in cardiac output. Doses of epidural lidocaine which produce blood levels in excess of 4 $\mu g.ml^{-1}$ caused hypotension owing in part to the negative inotropic action of lidocaine and the peripheral vasodilator effect of this agent.

Specific agents

Differences in the onset of epidural anaesthesia occur as a function of the specific agent employed and the concentration used. In general, local anaesthetics commonly used for epidural blockade can be classified as agents of rapid and slow onset. Chloroprocaine, lidocaine, mepivacaine, prilocaine and etidocaine produce a fairly rapid onset of anaesthesia, while bupivacaine is relatively slow in onset. With all agents there is a tendency for onset to be faster as the concentration is increased. The more rapidly acting agents tend to produce a more profound degree of hypotension due to the more rapid blockade of sympathetic fibres. In addition, certain agents such as etidocaine can penetrate myelinated fibres more readily and again may be associated with a more profound degree of sympathetic blockade and hypotension.

Addition of vasoconstrictors

Epinephrine is frequently added to local anaesthetics intended for epidural use in order to decrease the rate of vascular absorption and prolong the duration of anaesthesia. Absorbed epinephrine itself may produce transient cardiovascular alterations. A more profound degree of hypotension has been reported to occur following the use of epinephrine-containing local anaesthetics for epidural blockade. The absorbed epinephrine is believed to stimulate β_2-adrenergic receptors in all peripheral vascular beds, leading to an enhanced state of vasodilation and a fall in diastolic pressure. The β_1-adrenergic receptor stimulating effect of epinephrine results in an increase in heart rate and cardiac output which will counteract the peripheral vasodilator state to some extent. Although absorbed epinephrine may be responsible for the early cardiovascular changes observed following epidural block, the more prolonged hypotension seen with local anaesthetics containing epinephrine is probably related to the achievement of a more profound degree of sympathetic blockade.

Blood volume status

The cardiovascular alterations described above relate primarily to changes occurring in normovolaemic subjects. Cardiovascular depression is more severe and more dangerous following the production of epidural anaesthesia in hypovolaemic subjects. Epidural anaesthesia in mildly hypovolaemic volunteers was found to provoke vasovagal attacks associated with profound hypotension and bradycardia. Hypovolaemia is usually accompanied by compensatory vasoconstriction which will be abolished by the block, and cardiovascular collapse may ensue. The addition of epinephrine to the anaesthetic solution may result in a less profound degree of hypotension in hypovolaemic subjects. However, even the positive inotropic and chronotropic action of absorbed epinephrine cannot completely counteract the hypotensive effect of epidural blockade owing to the reduced circulating blood volume in these patients. Some authorities believe that hypovolaemia should be considered a relative contra-indication to the use of epidural anaesthesia unless adequate hydration or blood volume replacement is accomplished prior to the performance of the epidural block.

Effects on regional blood flow

The sympathetic nervous system plays an important part in regulating regional blood flow. Blockade of sympathetic nerve fibres and resulting loss of vasomotor tone will therefore cause considerable changes in the distribution of cardiac output, and epidural anaesthesia will produce significant changes in blood flow to various organs depending on the level of block achieved (Table 2:1). Investigations in monkeys utilizing a radioactive microsphere technique have shown that a T_{10} dermatomal level of anaesthesia resulted in an increase in lower limb blood flow but no significant changes in coronary, cerebral, renal or hepatic blood flow. High levels (T_1) of epidural block caused a 55% decrease in coronary blood flow. This decrease in coronary blood flow occurred concomitantly with a 47% decrease in mean arterial blood pressure. The decrease in myocardial work was greater than the decrease in coronary flow. Decreases in coronary blood flow have been observed in dogs following the intravenous administration of relatively large doses of lidocaine. Thus, the low coronary flows may be related in part to extensive sympathetic block or to the peripheral vasodilatory effect of lidocaine, both of which will cause systemic hypotension and decreased coronary perfusion.

Table 2:1
Effects of Epidural Anaesthesia on Regional Blood Flow

	Maximum % Decrease	
	T_5 level	T_1 level
Mean Arterial Pressure	20	45
Cardiac Output	10	30
Coronary Flow	25	55
Cerebral Flow	20	35
Hepatic Flow	20	40
Renal Flow	25	35

A significant decrease in cerebral blood flow of approximately 35% was also observed following achievement of a T_1 dermatomal level of epidural anaesthesia. Normally, cerebral blood flow is maintained constant owing to autoregulation, but below a critical arterial pressure the blood flow decreases and is compensated for by increased oxygen extraction from the arterial blood.

Renal blood flow also decreased significantly following attainment of a T_1 level of epidural anaesthesia in the monkey studies. A 31%-37% decrease in renal blood flow occurred at the time when mean arterial blood pressure and cardiac output were markedly reduced, suggesting that renal autoregulation also may be affected by a high epidural block.

Significant decreases in total hepatic blood flow of 20%-40% were observed following achievement of a T_1 level of anaesthesia. These changes in hepatic blood flow followed a 14%-47% decrease in mean arterial pressure.

Limited studies have been conducted in man with regard to regional blood flow during epidural anaesthesia. A 14% decrease in renal blood flow was observed in volunteers when a T_5 level of epidural blockade was produced. This change in renal blood flow occurred despite the lack of a significant decrease in mean arterial pressure and cardiac output. On the other hand hepatic blood flow changes during epidural anaesthesia in man parallel changes in mean arterial pressure.

The effect of epidural block on limb blood flow is predictable. A marked increase in blood flow in the lower limbs below the level of block is accompanied by a compensatory decrease in blood flow in upper limbs above the level of block. As a result, blood pressure may not change very much with a low level of epidural anaesthesia. However, high blocks will cause inhibition of sympathetic outflow to both upper and lower limbs, resulting in extensive vasodilation and a marked decrease in peripheral vascular resistance. Under these conditions limb blood flow will be directly related to the patient's blood pressure.

Metabolic and endocrine alterations

Nociceptive impulses which impinge on the hypothalamus and cerebral cortex result in the activation of efferent impulses to various endocrine organs. The endocrine and metabolic alterations which have been observed during surgery have led to the term "surgical stress", since the endocrine and metabolic changes are similar to those observed under a variety of stress situations.

Epidural anaesthesia itself appears to have little influence on endocrine function and metabolic activity. The induction of epidural anaesthesia prior to the start of surgery is not associated with any major changes in plasma levels of cortisol, prolactin, luteal hormone, follicular stimulating hormone or growth hormone. However, a decrease in plasma epinephrine and norepinephrine levels has been reported following the onset of epidural anaesthesia and studies with spinal anaesthesia suggest that changes in catecholamine plasma levels may be related to the level of block. Decreases in plasma epinephrine and norepinephrine can occur only if the block extends to the upper thoracic dermatomes.

With regard to metabolic products, epidural anaesthesia extending to the mid-thoracic level does not produce any significant changes in blood glucose, lactate, alanine, free fatty acids, glycerol and ketones. Data derived from spinal anaesthetic studies suggest that anaesthesia extending to upper thoracic dermatomal levels will inhibit the release of insulin which usually occurs in response to hyperglycaemia. Anaesthesia extending to the lower thoracic dermatomes failed to block the usual rise in insulin observed in response to hyperglycaemia.

Effect of epidural anaesthesia on surgically induced changes in endocrine and metabolic function

Surgical stimulation is associated with a variety of endocrine and metabolic changes (Tables 2:2, 2:3). These changes are related to an increase in metabolism that occurs in surgical patients, leading to a state of negative nitrogen balance in the postoperative period. The stress of surgery results in an increase in plasma concentrations of cortisol, aldosterone, renin, vasopressin, growth hormone, epinephrine and norepinephrine. In terms of metabolic alter-

Table 2:2
Effect of Epidural Anaesthesia on Surgically Induced Changes in Endocrine Functions

Endocrine Parameters	Surgery	Epidural Blockade
A. Pituitary hormones		
Prolactin	↑	Inhibit
Growth hormone	↑	Inhibit
ACTH	↑	Inhibit
ADH	↑	Inhibit
B. Adrenal and renal hormones		
Cortisol	↑	Inhibit
Aldosterone	↑	Inhibit
Renin	↑	Inhibit
Epinephrine	↑	Inhibit
Norepinephrine	↑	Inhibit
C. Pancreatic hormones		
Insulin	–	↓
Glucagon	–	–
D. Thyroid hormones		
Thyroxine	–	–
Triiodothyronine	↓	–

ations, increases in plasma glucose and lactate levels are usually seen following the start of surgery. Most of these surgically induced changes in endocrine and metabolic activity can be inhibited by adequate afferent blockade. However, procedures outside the area of block, such as endotracheal intubation, can provoke such changes. In addition it should be emphasised that to obtain the maximum modification of surgical stress the epidural block must be maintained well into the postoperative period.

Table 2:3
Effect of Epidural Anaesthesia on Surgically Induced Changes in Metabolic Functions

Metabolic Variables	Surgery	Epidural Blockade
Glucose	↑	Inhibit
Lactate	↑	Inhibit
3-hydroxybutyrate	↑	Inhibit
Glycerol	↑	Inhibit
Free fatty acids	↑	Inhibit
Alanine	↓	-
Cyclic AMP	↑	Inhibit

Pituitary hormones

Epidural anaesthesia can block the increase in plasma prolactin, growth hormone, ACTH and antidiuretic hormone. The inhibitory effect of epidural anaesthesia on these various pituitary hormonal levels may be related to the level of blockade and the site of surgery. For example, plasma ADH levels were inhibited by epidural anaesthesia during surgical procedures involving hip replacements. However, epidural anaesthesia extending to the mid-thoracic level failed to alter changes in plasma ADH observed following upper abdominal surgical procedures, presumably due to unblocked autonomic afferents in the vagus nerves and to endotracheal intubation.

Adrenal and renal hormones

Epidural anaesthesia can inhibit the surgically induced increase in plasma cortisol, aldosterone, renin, epinephrine, and norepinephrine. Again, the extent of the epidural blockade and the site of surgery will influence the degree of inhibition of these various hormones. Inhibition of plasma cortisol has consistently been observed in those patients undergoing epidural anaesthesia for lower abdominal surgical procedures such as hysterectomies or lower limb orthopaedic procedures. Little effect on the cortisol response to surgery has been observed when upper abdominal surgical procedures are performed. Similarly, little change in aldosterone and renin levels has been reported following epidural anaesthesia extending to the upper thoracic dermatomes for lower abdominal procedures. Other studies have failed to observe an inhibitory effect of epidural anaesthesia on the release of renin and aldosterone during surgical procedures performed in the upper abdomen, such as cholecystectomy. As indicated previously, epidural anaesthesia has been reported to inhibit increases in catecholamine levels observed during surgery. However, studies performed during spinal anaesthesia have suggested that this inhibitory effect is related to the level of blockade. Anaesthetic levels involving lower thoracic dermatomes failed to inhibit the rise in catecholamine levels, while those extending to the upper thoracic dermatomes were associated with inhibition of catecholamine elevations.

Pancreatic hormones

A decrease in plasma insulin levels has been observed following surgery performed under epidural anaesthesia, whereas there was little or no change in plasma glucagon. Glucose tolerance is much less affected by surgery if epidural rather than general anaesthesia is employed.

Thyroid hormones

Epidural anaesthesia does not appear to exert a significant influence on changes in plasma thyroxine and plasma tri-iodothyronine levels during surgery.

Metabolic alterations

The increase in plasma glucose usually observed following the start of surgery can be effectively inhibited by epidural anaesthesia. Epidural anaesthesia has also been shown to inhibit the surgically related increase in blood lactate and 3-hydroxybutyrate. In terms of fat metabolism, surgical procedures involving the lower abdomen performed under epidural anaesthesia are associated with decreased levels of plasma glycerol and free fatty acids. Upper abdominal surgical procedures or analgesia extending only to the lower thoracic dermatomes have not been associated with similar changes in free fatty acids.

The mechanism by which epidural anaesthesia may inhibit endocrine changes and metabolic alterations during surgery is probably related to a blockade of either afferent or efferent pathways or both. The ability of epidural anaesthesia to inhibit the release of pituitary hormones is probably due to the blockade of afferent nociceptive pathways. On the other hand, the inhibition of the release of adrenal cortical hormones such as cortisol may result from an inhibition of efferent pathways or, more likely, from the inhibition of the release of ACTH from the pituitary gland during afferent blockade. Inhibition of the release of catecholamines from the adrenal medulla is probably related to the blockade of efferent autonomic pathways by epidural anaesthesia. Similarly, the decrease in the release of insulin from the pancreas is probably due to the blockade of efferent sympathetic fibres to the pancreas.

The inhibition of the hyperglycaemic response to surgery by epidural anaesthesia may be related in part to the blockade of efferent sympathetic nerves to the liver and also the inhibition of epinephrine release from the adrenal medulla. The combination of efferent sympathetic blockade and inhibition of epinephrine release will result in a decreased rate of glycogenolysis in the liver during surgery. Although the hyperglycaemic response to surgery is inhibited by epidural anaesthesia, intravenous glucose tolerance tests performed during surgery under epidural anaesthesia are essentially normal. This may be related to the decrease in the rate of glycogenolysis during epidural anaesthesia, the inhibition of the rise in cortisol and epinephrine levels during surgical procedures performed under epidural anaesthesia, and the failure of epidural anaesthesia to alter the insulin response to hyperglycaemia.

The failure of epidural anaesthesia to inhibit the endocrine-metabolic stress response for upper abdominal surgical procedures or in situations in which the spread of epidural anaesthesia is inadequate, is believed to be due to the inability to block afferent pathways conducted through the vagus nerve. However, studies in which the vagus nerves were inhibited by local infiltration with local anaesthetics failed to demonstrate a blockade of the increase in cortisol blood levels observed during surgery in the upper abdominal area carried out under epidural anaesthesia. Thus, the inability to block afferent pathways in the vagus may not be responsible for the lack of effect of epidural anaesthesia in certain surgical situations. The failure to block all afferent pathways by a seemingly adequate epidural anaesthetic is not understood. The observation of missed segments following the performance of a routine epidural anaesthetic procedure in labour suggests that all nociceptive afferent pathways may not be adequately blocked by epidural anaesthesia. Thus, the stress associated with an upper abdominal surgical procedure may be sufficiently great that it is difficult for an epidurally administered local anaesthetic to inhibit completely all nociceptive afferent pathways.

References & Bibliography

Bonica, J.J., Berges, P.U., and Morikawa, K. (1971). Circulatory effects of peridural block I. Effects of levels of analgesia and dose of lidocaine. Anesthesiology 33:619.

Bonica, J.J., Akamatsu, T.J., Berges, P.U. and Kennedy, W.F. (1972). Circulatory effects of peridural block II. Effects of epinephrine. Anesthesiology 34:514.

Bonica, J.J., Kennedy, W.F., Akamatsu, T.J. and Gerbershagen, J.U. (1972). Circulatory effects of peridural block III. Effects of acute blood loss. Anesthesiology 36:219.

Bromage, P.R., Joyal, A.C. and Binney, J.C. (1963). Local anesthetic drugs. Penetration from the spinal extradural space into the neuraxis. Science 140:392.

Bromage, P.R. (1978): Epidural Analgesia. Philadelphia. W.B. Saunders Company.

Bromage, P.R. (1975): Mechanism of action of extradural analgesia. Brit. J. Anaesth. 47:199.

Cohan, E.N. (1968). Distribution of local anesthetic agents in the neuraxis of the dog. Anesthesiology 29:1002.

Cusick, J.F., Myklebust, J.B. and Abram, S.E. (1980): Differential neural effects of epidural anesthetics. Anesthesiology 53:299.

Frumin, M.J., Schwartz, H. and Burns, J.J., Brodie, B.B., and Papper, E.M. (1953). The appearnce of procaine in the spinal fluid during peridural block in man. J. Pharmacol. Exp. Ther. 109:102.

Gasser, H.S. and Erlanger, J. (1980). The role of fiber size in the establishment of a nerve block by pressure or cocaine. Am. J. Physiol. 88:581.

Gissen, A.J., Covino, B.G., Gregus, J. (1980). Differential sensitivities of mammalian nerve fibers to local anesthetic agents. Anesthesiology 53:467.

Gissen, A.J., Covino, B.G., Gregus, J. (1982). Differential sensitivity of fast and slow fibers in mammalian nerve II. Margin of safety for nerve transmission. Anesth. Analg. 61:561.

Kehlet, H., Brandt, M.R., Hansen, A.P. and Alberti, K.G.M.M. (1979). Effect of epidural analgesia on metabolic profiles during and after surgery. Br. J. Surg. 66:543.

Kehlet, H. (1982): The modifying effect of general and regional anesthesia on the endocrine-metabolic response to surgery. Reg. Anesth. 7:S38.

Melzack, R. and Wall, P.D. (1965). Pain mechanisms: A new theory. Science 150:971.

Rexed, B. (1954). The cytoarchitectonic atlas of the spinal cord in the cat. J. Comp. Nuerol. 100:297.

Scott, D.B., Littlewood, D.G., Drummond, G.B., Buckley, B.F. and Covino, B.G. (1977). Modification of the circulatory effects of extradural block combined with general anaesthesia by the addition of adrenaline to lignocaine solutions. Brit. J. Anaesth. 49:917.

Shantha, T.R. and Evans, J.A. (1972). The relationship of epidural anesthesia to neural membranes and arachnoid villi. Anesthesiology 37:543.

Sivarajan, M., Amory, D.W. and Lindbloom, L.E. (1976). Systemic and regional blood flow during epidural anesthesia without epinephrine in the rhesus monkey. Anesthesiology 45:300

Stanton-Hicks, M., Murphy, T.M., Bonica, J.J., Berges, P.U., Mather, L.E. and Tucker, G.T. (1975). Effects of peridural block: V. Properties, circulatory effects, and blood levels of etidocaine and lidocaine. Anesthesiology 42:398.

3. Pharmacological considerations

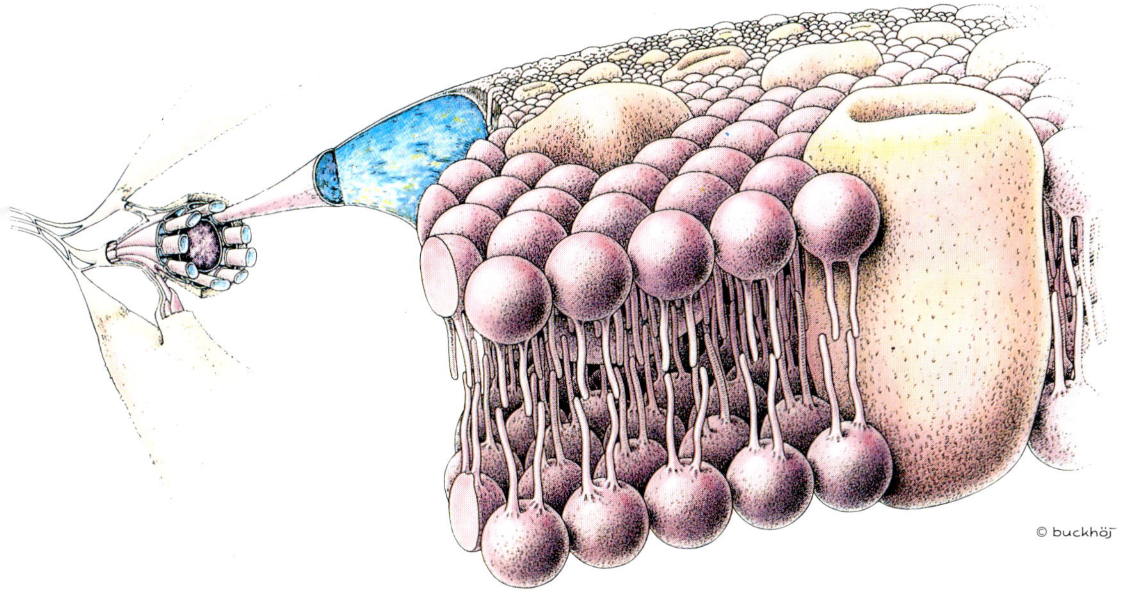

Local anaesthetic agents

Local anaesthetic drugs are chemical compounds whose primary pharmacological activity involves inhibition of the excitation conduction process in peripheral nerves. Like many of the early therapeutic agents, the first local anaesthetic, cocaine, was a naturally occurring alkaloid that had been isolated from the leaves of the Erythroxylon coca bush, which was indigenous to South America. The introduction of cocaine into clinical practice has been attributed to Koller, who described the topical anaesthetic properties of this agent for ophthalmological use in 1884. However, both the anaesthetic and the CNS stimulant activity of cocaine had been recognised by the South American natives for many years prior to Koller's presentation. Procaine was synthesised by Einhorn in 1905 and represented the first safe injectable agent of clini-

Fig. 3:1 Relationship between nerve action potential and movement of sodium and potassium ions across the nerve membrane. a. At rest an excess of sodium ions (green dots) are present on the outside of nerve membrane and an excess of potassium ions (blue dots) are present on the inside of the nerve membrane. b. During the depolarization phase of the action potential, sodium ions flow from the outside to the inside of the nerve membrane through open sodium channels. c. During the repolarization phase of the action potential, the sodium channels close and potassium ions flow through open potassium channels from the inside to the outside of the membrane. d. At the conclusion of the action potential, sodium and potassium ions are actively transported back to their original position as in fig. 3:1a.

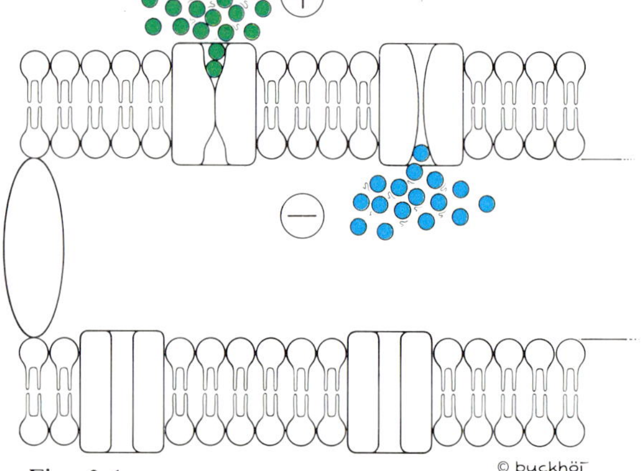

Fig. 3:1a

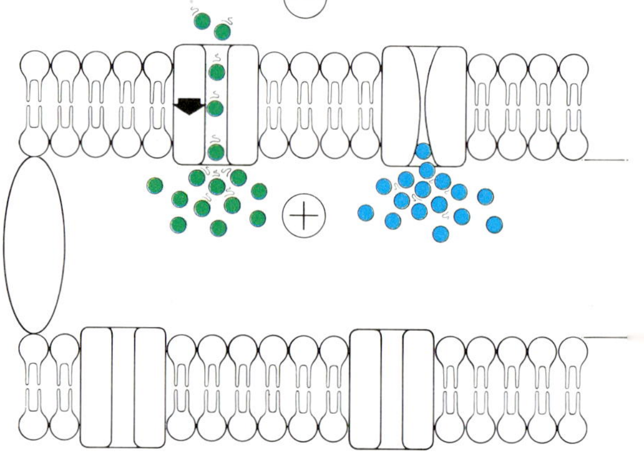

Fig. 3:1b

cal value for the production of local anaesthesia. Following the introduction of procaine, numerous compounds of similar chemical structure were developed. Tetracaine and chloroprocaine are the procaine-like agents which have persisted to this day as clinically useful local anaesthetics.

In 1943, Löfgren synthesised lidocaine, which represented a new chemical class of local anaesthetic compounds. Whereas the procaine-like drugs are ester derivatives of para-aminobenzoic acid, lidocaine is an amide derivative of diethylamino-acetic acid. Since the advent of lidocaine, many other amide substances such as mepivacaine, prilocaine, bupivacaine and etidocaine have been introduced into clinical practice as local anaesthetic agents, each with its own pharmacological profile.

Mechanism of local anaesthesia

The conduction of impulses along nerve fibres is related to changes in the electrical gradient across the nerve membrane which, in turn, are a function of the movement of certain ions, particularly sodium and potassium, across the membrane (Fig. 3:1a, b, c and d). A stimulus of sufficient intensity will reduce the resting membrane potential from approximately -90 mV to approximately -60 mV, i.e. the threshold potential level following which a spontaneous rapid phase of depolarisation will occur. Depolarisation in one segment of an unmyelinated nerve will result in depolarisation in the adjacent segment due to the difference in electrical potential between a depolarised and a polarised segment (Fig. 3:2). In this way, a stimulus applied to one end of a nerve will be transmitted the entire length of the nerve fibre. In myelinated nerves the impulse passes from one node of

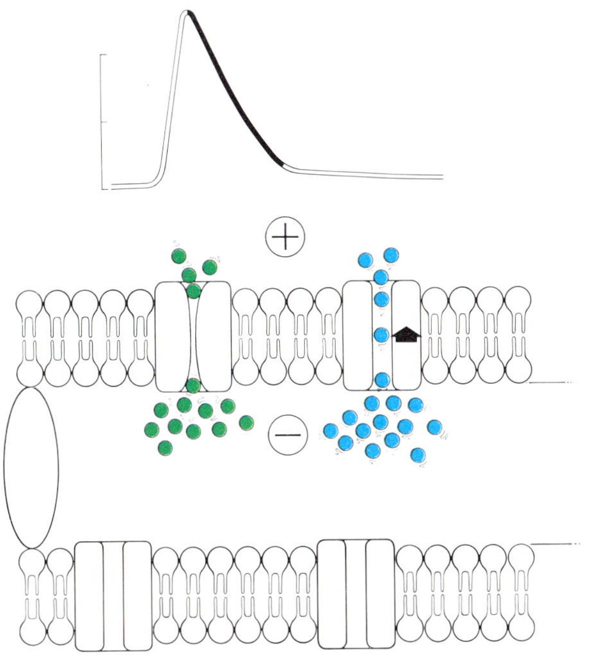

Fig. 3:1c

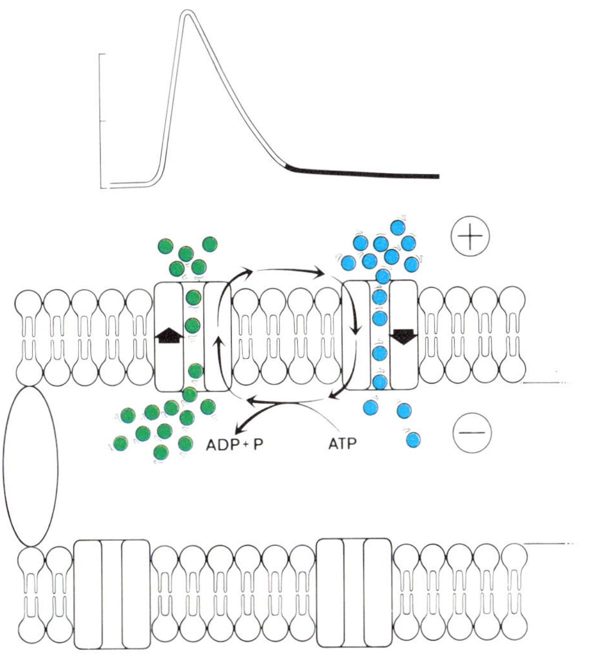

Fig. 3:1d

Ranvier to the adjacent node (Fig. 3:2). Repolarisation results in the return of the nerve membrane to the original resting potential level.

Depolarisation is due to the inward passage of sodium ions from the extracellular to the intracellular space by way of specific sodium channels in the membrane. The flow of potassium ions from the interior to the exterior of the nerve is responsible for the repolarisation phase. At the completion of the action potential ionic equilibrium is re-established by the activation of the sodium-potassium pump in the nerve membrane (Fig. 3:1d). Local anaesthetic agents prevent depolarisation of the nerve membrane by inhibiting the flow of sodium ions (Fig. 3:1b). Direct measurements of sodium and potassium conductance in the giant squid axon by voltage clamp techniques have shown that conventional local anaesthetics primarly block sodium currents, while having minimal effects on potassium currents. For example, 20 $mM.l^{-1}$ of lidocaine causes complete inhibition of sodium conductance but only a 5% decrease in potassium conductance. In addition, tetradotoxin, the puffer fish poison, completely blocks sodium conductance and electrical conduction in nerves, with no discernible effect on potassium conductance. These studies clearly indicate that inhibition of sodium conductance is basically responsible for conduction blockade by local anaesthetic drugs.

It has been postulated by some investigators that the inhibition of sodium flux is mediated by an interaction between the local anaesthetic and calcium. Local anaesthetic activity is enhanced in the presence of low calcium and an increase in the calcium ion concentration can reverse the conduction block induced by the application of local anaesthetic agents to isolated nerves. Local anaesthetics have also been shown to accelerate the release of calcium from skeletal muscle. Finally, in vitro studies have demonstrated that local anaesthetics are capable of inhibiting the binding of calcium to phosphatidyl-l-serine and that a

Fig. 3.2 a. and b. Propagation of a nerve impulse along myelinated and unmyelinated nerve fibres. a. Impulse passes from one node of Ranvier to the next in myelinated nerve fibres. b. Impulse passes along the entire length of the unmyelinated nerve.

a.

b.

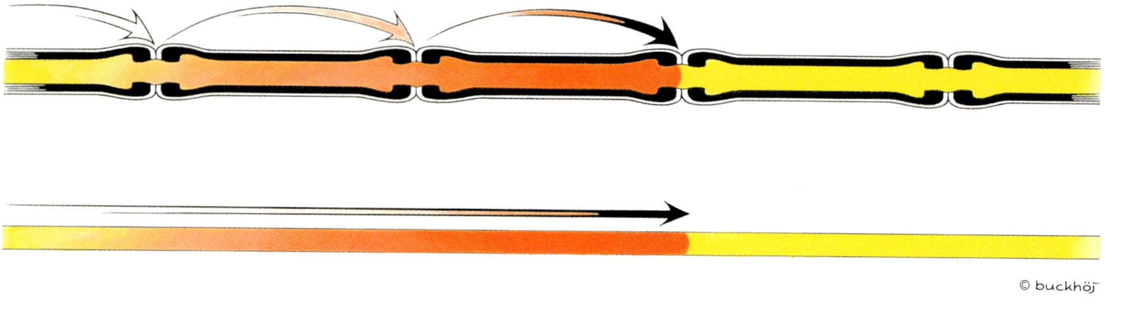

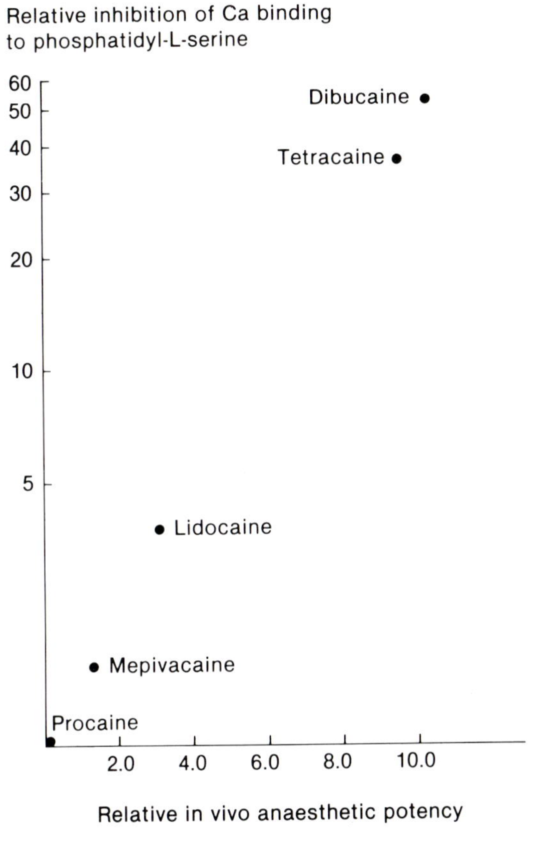

Fig. 3.3 Relationship between the inhibition of calcium binding to phosphatidyl-l-serine and the relative anaesthetic potency of various agents.

Fig. 3:4 Diagram of the structure of the nerve membrane which consists of a lipid bilayer and protein molecules which contain the sodium channels.

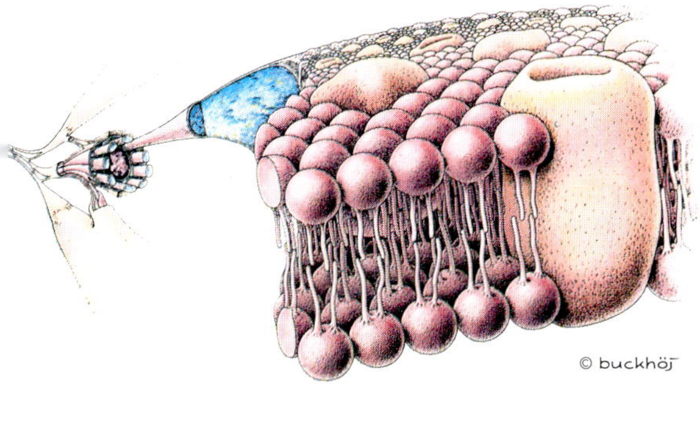

correlation exists between their ability to do this and their anaesthetic potency (Fig. 3:3). Although calcium can antagonise the effect of local anaesthetic agents, more recent studies have indicated that calcium does not alter the inhibitory effect of local anaesthetics on sodium conductance, suggesting that the actions of both calcium and local anaesthetics occur at different sites in the nerve membrane. At present calcium is not believed to mediate the action of local anaesthetic agents on sodium conductance.

The site of action of local anaesthetic agents undoubtedly involves the sodium channels in the nerve membrane. The membrane is a lipoprotein matrix (Fig. 3:4). Conventional local anaesthetics such as lidocaine diffuse through the membrane to the axoplasm and then enter the sodium channels, where they interact with specific receptors (Fig. 3:5).

Fig. 3:5 Passage of local anaesthetic molecules across the nerve membrane and entering a sodium channel from the axoplasmic surface.

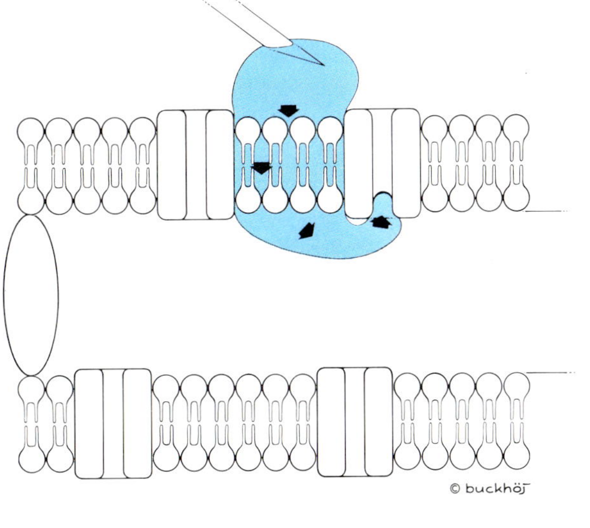

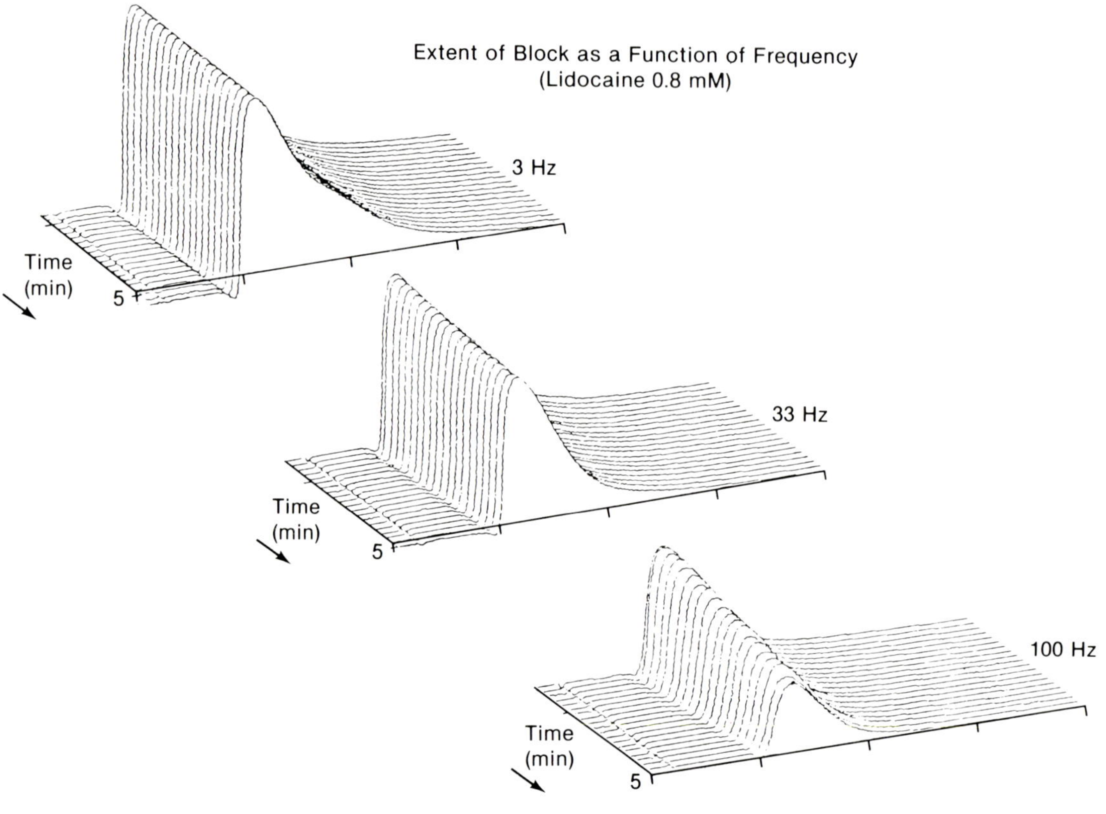

Fig. 3:6 Relationship between depression of action potential amplitude and frequency of nerve stimulation in the presence of lidocaine.

Fig. 3:7 Various states of the sodium channel. (1) closed. (2) open. (3) inactivated.

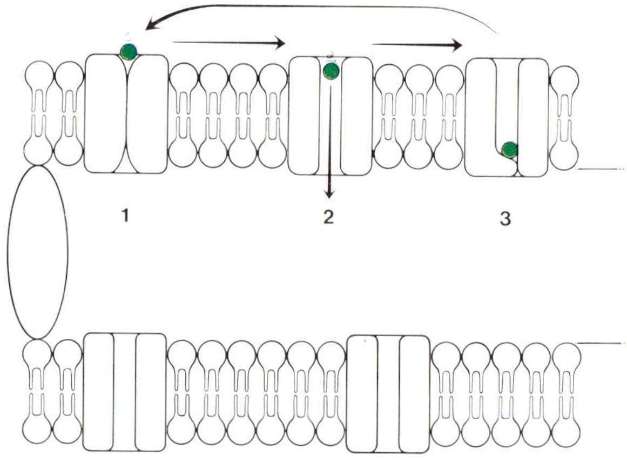

Studies involving frequency-dependent conduction blockade also implicate the interior of the sodium channel as the site for binding of local anaesthetics to a receptor. For example, the degree of action potential suppression by agents such as lidocaine is directly correlated with the frequency of nerve stimulation (Fig. 3:6). This phenomenon is related to the time during which the sodium channels are in an open state. The sodium channels in the nerve membrane are believed to exist in three states: closed, open and inactive (Fig. 3:7). At rest the channels exist in a closed state such that neither sodium ions nor drugs enter the channels. Application of an appropriate stimulus to a nerve will open the channel, allowing the passage of sodium ions and also allowing drugs such as local anaesthetics to gain access to the interior of the channel from the axoplasm. Upon completion of the depolarisation phase, the channel passes through an inactive state before returning to the resting closed state. As the frequency of stimulation is increased, the sodium channels remain in an open state for a longer period. Therefore, the local anaesthetic agent which has diffused across the membrane into the axoplasm will have a greater opportunity to penetrate the interior of the sodium channel when the nerve is being stimulated at a higher frequency.

Other mechanisms for conduction blockade may also exist. As will be discussed later, the ionised form of a conventional local anaesthetic is believed to bind to a receptor site in the sodium channel to cause conduction block. However, benzocaine and benzyl alcohol are compounds which exist only in a non-ionised form and yet possess local anaesthetic activity. Conduction block produced by these agents can be reversed by high atmospheric pressures, whereas the effect of conventional local anaesthetics is only partially reversed following exposure of nerves to high pressures. Moreover, the anaesthetic potency of these neutral agents is related to the amount of drug taken up by the nerve membrane, which, in turn, is a function of the lipid solubility of the drugs. Based on these observations, agents such as benzocaine and benzyl alcohol are believed to inhibit sodium flux and block nerve conduction by an expansion or alteration in the configuration of the nerve membrane, which will decrease the diameter of the sodium channel (Fig. 3:8). In essence, these agents are believed to act in a fashion similar to the general anaesthetics.

Finally, the biotoxins, tetradotoxin and saxitoxin, are extremely potent local anaesthetics whose sites of action are apparently different from those of the conventional agents and the neutral compounds. These biotoxins, which exist only in a charged form, do not readily penetrate nerve membranes. In addition, they do not inhibit conduction when applied to the axoplasmic surface of the nerve. However, they are very potent anaesthetics when placed on the external surface of the nerve, indicating that they inhibit sodium conductance and cause conduction block by an action on the external surface of the sodium channel.

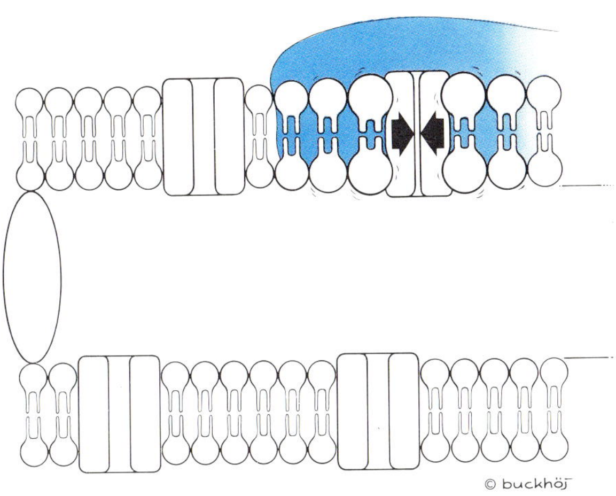

Fig. 3:8 Agents such as benzocaine decrease diameter of the sodium channel by membrane expansion or alteration in the configuration of the nerve membrane.

Summarising, three distinct sites of action have been proposed for various chemical compounds which possess local anaesthetic activity (Fig. 3:9). The biotoxins are believed to combine with a receptor site at the external opening of the sodium channel. Conventional local anaesthetic agents interact with a receptor site at the internal opening of the sodium channel. Compounds such as benzocaine penetrate the nerve membrane and cause conformational changes which lead to a decrease in the diameter of the sodium channel. This membrane expansion can also occur when the basic forms of conventional agents are within the membrane (see below).

In an in vivo situation, diffusion of local anaesthetics to their site of action is also an important consideration with regard to the mechanism of local anaesthesia. Diffusion is related to the degree of ionisation of the various agents. In solution the clinically useful local anaesthetic agents exist both in the form of uncharged molecules and as positively charged cations. The relative proportion between the uncharged base and the charged cation depends on the pK_a of the specific chemical compound and the pH of the solution. Since pK_a is constant for any specific compound, the relative proportion of free base and charged cation would be dependent essentially on the pH of the local anaesthetic solution. As the pH of the solution is decreased, equilibrium will shift towards the charged cationic form and relatively more cation will be present than free base. Conversely, as the pH is increased, the equilibrium will shift towards the free base form. Because the pH of commercially available local anaesthetic solutions is essentially dependent on the solubility of the local anaesthetic substance, the ability to alter the pH over wide ranges and thus influence the amount of drug in the base or charged cationic form is limited.

Both the uncharged base form and the

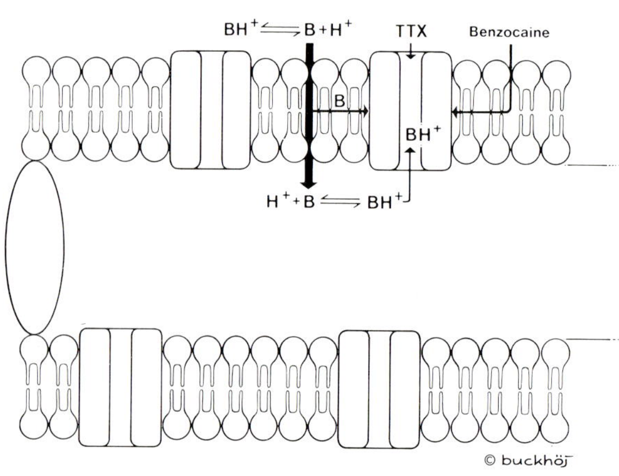

Fig. 3:9 Various sites of action for different types of local anaesthetic agents. Biotoxins such as tetradotoxin (TTX) act at the external surface of sodium channels. Conventional local anaesthetics (B) such as lidocaine act at the axoplasmic surface of the sodium channels, and to some extent by membrane expansion. Agents such as benzocaine act by membrane expansion.

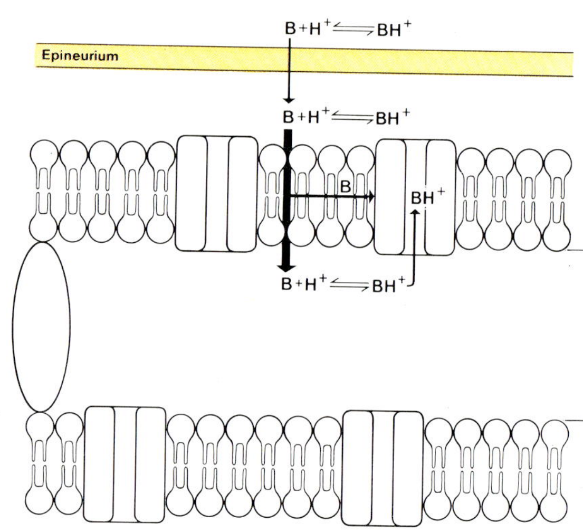

Fig. 3:10 Diffusion of local anaesthetic agents across nerve sheath and membrane to the receptor site. The base form (B) diffuses most readily across the nerve sheath and nerve membrane. The ionized form (BH+) which appears when the base form reaches the axoplasm, then attaches to the receptor site in the sodium channels.

charged cationic form of local anaesthetic agents are involved in the process of conduction blockade. Only the base diffuses through the nerve sheath and is therefore required for optimal penetration of the local anaesthetic into the axoplasm, where equilibrium reoccurs between the base and cationic forms (Fig. 3:10). It is the charged cation which actually binds to the receptor site in the sodium channel and is ultimately responsible for the inhibition of sodium conductance. Although the cationic form plays the major role in conduction blockade by the clinically useful local anaesthetic agents, the free base may contribute to the local anaesthetic activity by causing expansion of the nerve membrane in a fashion similar to that of benzocaine. The ability of high atmospheric pressure to partially reverse the blockade produced by local anaesthetic agents, such as procaine and lidocaine, suggests that the base form may exert some blocking activity by virtue of its ability to slightly expand the nerve membrane.

In summary, the sequence of events which results in conduction blockade in peripheral nerves by conventional local anaesthetic agents is as follows:

1. Diffusion of the base form across the nerve sheath and nerve membrane.

2. Re-equilibration between the base and cationic forms in the axoplasm.

3. Penetration of the cation into and attachment to a receptor at a site within the sodium channel.

4. Blockade of the sodium channel.

5. Inhibition of sodium conductance.

6. Decrease in the rate and degree of the depolarization phase of the action potential.

7. Failure to achieve the threshold potential.

8. Lack of development of a propagated action potential.

9. Conduction blockade.

Structure-activity relationship of local anaesthetic agents

Chemical compounds that demonstrate local anaesthetic activity usually possess an aromatic and an amine group separated by an intermediate chain (Table 3:1). The clinically useful local anaesthetic agents essentially fall into one of two chemically distinct groups. Those agents which possess an ester link between the aromatic portion and the intermediate chain are referred to as amino esters and include procaine, chloroprocaine and tetracaine. Local anaesthetics with an amide link between the aromatic end and the intermediate chain are referred to as amino amides and include lidocaine, mepivacaine, prilocaine, bupivacaine and etidocaine. The basic difference between the ester and the amide compounds resides in their chemical stability. Esters are easily hydrolysed and are relatively unstable in solution. Amides, on the other hand, arc not hydrolysed and are much more stable. In

Table 3:1
Physicochemical Properties of Local Anaesthetics

Agent	Aromatic Lipophilic	Intermediate Chain	Amine Hydrophilic	Molecular Weight (base)	pKa (25°C)	Partition Coefficient	Per Cent Protein Binding
Esters							
Procaine	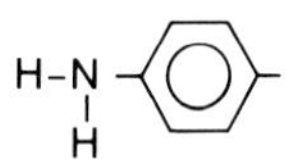	$COOCH_2CH_2$	$-N(C_2H_5)_2$	236	8.9	0.02	5.8
Tetracaine	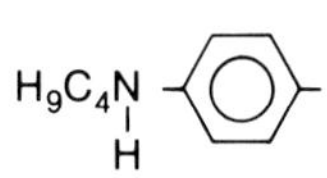	$COOCH_2CH_2$	$-N(CH_3)_2$	264	8.6	4.1	75.6
Chloroprocaine	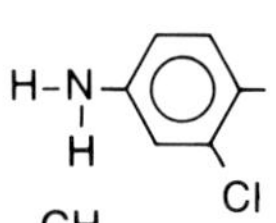	$COOCH_2CH_2$	$-N(C_2H_5)_2$	271	8.7	0.14	-
Amides							
Prilocaine	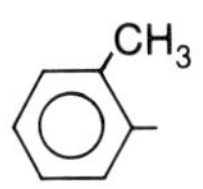	$NHCOCH(CH_3)$	$-N(H)(C_3H_7)$	220	7.7	0.9	55 approx.
Lidocaine	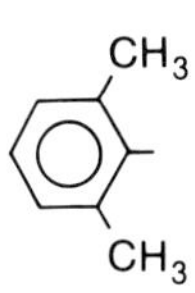	$NHCOCH_2$	$-N(C_2H_5)_2$	234	7.7	2.9	64.3
Mepivacaine		NHCO	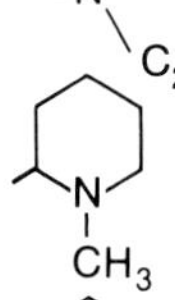	246	7.6	0.8	77.5
Bupivacaine		NHCO	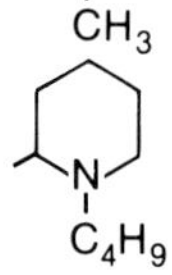	288	8.1	27.5	95.6
Etidocaine		$NHCOCH(C_2H_5)$	$-N(C_2H_5)(C_3H_7)$	276	7.7	141	94

the body, the amino esters are hydrolysed in plasma by the enzyme cholinesterase, whereas the amide compounds undergo enzymatic degradation in the liver. Para-aminobenzoic acid is one of the metabolites formed from the hydrolysis of ester type compounds, and this substance is capable of inducing allergic type reactions in a small percentage of patients. The amino amides, however, are not metabolised to para-aminobenzoic acid, and reports of allergic reactions to these agents are extremely rare.

The clinically important properties of local anaesthetic agents include potency, speed of onset and duration of anaesthetic activity. These properties are essentially determined by the physicochemical characteristics of the various compounds, which in turn are dependent on their chemical structure. The properties which influence anaesthetic activity are lipid solubility, protein binding and pK_a. Minor changes in molecular structure have dramatic effects on these properties (Table 3:1).

Lipid solubility appears to be the primary determinant of intrinsic anaesthetic potency, whereas protein binding appears related to the duration of anaesthetic activity. Consideration of the biochemical composition of the nerve membrane provides a logical explanation for the importance of lipid solubility and protein binding as determinants of anaesthetic potency and duration. The nerve membrane is basically a lipoprotein matrix (Fig. 3:4). The axolemma consists of 90% lipids and 10% proteins. As a result, chemical compounds which are highly lipophilic tend to penetrate the nerve membrane more easily, such that fewer molecules are required for conduction blockade, resulting in enhanced potency. In general, receptors involved in drug action are believed to be protein in nature. Therefore, local anaesthetic agents which have a high affinity for the receptor protein in the sodium channel will tend to remain at the receptor site for a prolonged period of time, resulting in an extended duration of anaesthetic activity. A correlation does exist between the lipid solubility and protein binding of local anaesthetics and their inherent potency and duration.

The pK_a of a chemical compound is the pH at which the ionised and non-ionised forms are present in equal amounts. Since the uncharged form of the local anaesthetic agent is primarily responsible for diffusion across the nerve sheath and nerve membrane, the onset of action will be directly related to the amount of drug which exists in the base form. The percentage of a specific local anaesthetic drug which is present in the base form when injected into tissue, whose pH is 7.4, is inversely proportional to the pK_a of that agent. For example, mepivacaine, lidocaine, prilocaine and etidocaine possess a pK_a of approximately 7.7. When these agents are injected into tissue they are rapidly buffered to a pH of 7.4. At this physiological pH approximately 65% of these drugs exists in the ionised form and 35% in the non-ionised base form. On the other hand, tetracaine possesses a pK_a of 8.6, and only 5% is present in the non-ionised form at a tissue pH of 7.4, while 95% exists in the charged cationic form.

The pK_a of bupivacaine is 8.1, which means that 20% of this agent is present in the non-ionised form at a tissue pH of 7.4, and 80% exists in the charged cationic form. Studies on isolated nerves have shown that the onset of conduction blockade is related to the pK_a of the local anaesthetic (Table 3:2). Lidocaine, prilocaine and etidocaine show a rapid onset of action whereas procaine, with a high pK_a, has a slow onset time.

The anaesthetic characteristics of various chemical compounds in vivo are dependent in part on other miscellaneous considerations. The onset of action may be altered by the rate of diffusion through non-nervous tissue. For example, lidocaine and prilocaine possess a similar pK_a and similar onset of action in an isolated nerve. However, in vivo studies suggest that prilocaine may be somewhat slower in onset than lidocaine. This difference may be related to an enhanced ability of lidocaine to diffuse through non-nervous tissue. More important, nevertheless, is the concentration of local anaesthetic agent employed. For example, 0.25% bupivacaine possesses a rather slow onset of action. However, increasing the concentration to 0.75% results in a significant decrease in the latency of anaesthetic activity. The rapid onset time of chloroprocaine in vivo may be related in part to improved diffusion through non-nervous tissue, but also to the use of a 3% concentration of this agent. The pK_a of chloroprocaine is approximately 9 and its onset of action in isolated nerves is relatively slow. However, the low systemic toxicity of this agent allows the use of high concentrations. Therefore, the rapid onset time in vivo of chloroprocaine may be related simply to the large number of molecules placed in the vicinity of peripheral nerves.

The effect of local anaesthetic agents on the vasculature at the site of injection will also influence the in vivo potency and duration of action of these compounds. Absorption of local anaesthetic agents from the region of their injection will decrease the number of molecules available for diffusion to the receptor site in the nerve membrane (Fig. 3:11). Factors which increase the absorption will decrease the apparent anaesthetic potency and duration of action of a specific compound. All local anaesthetics with the exception of cocaine exhibit a biphasic effect on vascular smooth muscle. At extremely low concentrations they cause enhanced activity of vascular smooth muscle, leading to vasoconstriction, while, in the concentrations commonly employed for regional anaesthesia, they tend to be vasodilators. The relative degree of vasodilation produced by different local anaesthetic drugs can affect their potency and duration of action. This can be demon-

Table 3:2
Relationship of pKa to Percent Base Form and Time for 50 Percent Conduction Block in Isolated Nerve

Agent	pKa	% Base at pH 7.4	Onset (min)
Prilocaine	7.7	35	2-4
Lidocaine	7.7	35	2-4
Etidocaine	7.7	35	2-4
Bupivacaine	8.1	20	5-8
Tetracaine	8.6	5	10-15
Procaine	8.9	2	14-18

Fig. 3:11 Following the injection of a local anaesthetic, a portion is absorbed by vascular beds in the area of the injection while the remainder diffuses either to the nerve fibres where conduction block occurs, or into epidural fat.

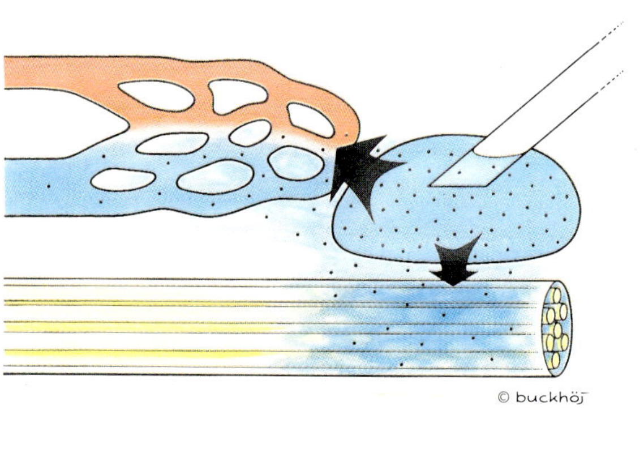

strated by comparing the in vitro and in vivo activity of different agents. For example, in vitro studies of lidocaine and mepivacaine have shown that lidocaine is significantly more potent than mepivacaine on an isolated nerve while the duration of conduction blockade is similar. However, in vivo studies have shown little difference in their relative anaesthetic potency and, indeed, the duration of action of mepivacaine is somewhat longer than that of lidocaine. These differences appear to be related to a greater degree of vasodilation produced by lidocaine. Addition of a vasoconstrictor agent such as epinephrine to solutions of both lidocaine and mepivacaine eliminates the difference in duration of the two compounds, which again suggests that the greater vasodilator activity of lidocaine is responsible for the difference in anaesthetic duration observed between the plain solutions.

The only agent which produces a state of vasoconstriction at clinically useful concentrations is cocaine. The vasoconstrictor action of cocaine is not directly related to the agent itself but is an indirect action. Cocaine possesses the ability to prevent the re-uptake of norepinephrine by storage granules which results in a state of vasoconstriction.

In summary, the pharmacological activity of local anaesthetic agents is related primarily to their physicochemical properties. However, the activity of these agents in vivo may be altered by other actions which are essentially unrelated to their physicochemical properties. On the basis of anaesthetic activity in man, the various agents may be classified as follows:

1. Agents of low anaesthetic potency and short duration of action: procaine and chloroprocaine.

2. Agents of intermediate anaesthetic potency and duration of action: lidocaine, mepivacaine and prilocaine.

3. Agents of high anaesthetic potency and prolonged duration of action: tetracaine, bupivacaine and etidocaine.

In terms of latency, chloroprocaine, lidocaine, mepivacaine, prilocaine and etidocaine possess a relatively rapid onset of action. Bupivacaine is intermediate in terms of onset of anaesthesia, while procaine and tetracaine demonstrate a long latency period.

Agents for epidural use

The local anaesthetics which may be used for epidural blockade are shown in Table 3:3. Procaine and tetracaine are rarely employed. Procaine has a slow onset, low potency and a relatively short duration of action. Tetracaine has a slow onset of action and a narrow safety margin. Chloroprocaine has enjoyed popularity in the United States as an epidural anaesthetic agent for obstetrical use. This agent is characterised by a rapid onset time and a wide therapeutic ratio in terms of systemic toxicity for mother and foetus. The very short duration of chloroprocaine limits its usefulness for surgical epidural anaesthesia. Recent evidence that chloroprocaine solutions have been associated with prolonged neurological deficits in some patients, following accidental administration of large quantities into the subarachnoid space, may also limit its use for epidural anaesthesia (see Chap. 6, p. 154).

Lidocaine, mepivacaine and prilocaine are similar in terms of their anaesthetic profile when used for epidural blockade. Lidocaine may possess a slightly shorter onset time, while mepivacaine and prilocaine produce a longer duration of anaesthesia than lidocaine when the agents are used without a vasoconstrictor. Prilocaine is systemically the least toxic of the various amide local anaesthetics. Unfortunately, doses above 600 mg are associated with the formation of methaemoglobinaemia, which has limited the use of this agent. Nevertheless, it is an excellent agent if such doses are not exceeded.

Bupivacaine and etidocaine are employed as epidural agents of relatively long duration. They differ considerably in their anaesthetic profile, although they are both potent, long-acting agents. Bupivacaine is widely used for both surgical and obstetrical epidural anaesthesia. It is of particular value for continuous epidural blockade during labour. When used as an 0.25% or 0.5% solution it provides satisfactory sensory analgesia with minimal motor blockade. Thus, the patient in labour can be rendered pain free and still be able to move her legs. In addition, bupivacaine usually provides 2-3 h of adequate analgesia, although this depends greatly on the dosage. The onset of anaesthesia is relatively slow, frequently requiring 15-20 min for development of an adequate epidural block. For surgical procedures the 0.75% concentration of bupivacaine appears more useful than the 0.25% or 0.5% solutions. The latency is shortened, the depth of analgesia is more profound and muscular relaxation is improved. However, 0.75% bupivacaine is no longer recommended for obstetrical anaesthesia owing to reports of severe cardiotoxic reactions (see Chap. 6, p. 150).

Table 3:3
Agents for Epidural Blockade

Agent	Usual Concentration	Usual Onset (min)	Usual Duration of Surg. Anaes.	Main Clinical Use
Chloroprocaine	2-3	5-15	30-90	Obstetrics
Lidocaine	1-2	5-15	60-120	Obstetrics Surgery
Mepivacaine	1-2	5-15	60-150	Surgery
Prilocaine	1-3	5-15	60-150	Surgery
Bupivacaine	0.25-0.75	10-20	120-240	Obstetrics Surgery
Etidocaine	1.0-1.5	5-15	120-240	Surgery

Etidocaine is especially useful for surgical procedures, including Caesarean sections. When used as a 1.5% solution this agent provides the most rapid onset of any local anaesthetic administered epidurally. Initial signs of analgesia appear in 3-5 min and may be complete in 10 min. Etidocaine shows little sensory/motor discrimination. Thus, dosages of this agent that provide satisfactory analgesia invariably produce profound motor blockade. In surgical situations where optimal muscle relaxation is desirable, etidocaine has proven to be a valuable agent for epidural use since it combines a rapid onset, duration of 3-4 h and a satisfactory quality of analgesia with profound muscle relaxation. However, this marked effect on motor function renders etidocaine of limited value for obstetrical analgesia as opposed to anaesthesia.

The use of mixtures of different local anaesthetics for epidural blockade has become relatively popular in recent years. The basis for this practice is to compensate for the short duration of action of certain agents such as chloroprocaine and the long latency of other agents such as tetracaine and bupivacaine. The combination of lidocaine or mepivacaine and tetracaine was commonly employed in some centres prior to the advent of bupivacaine and etidocaine as long duration anaesthetics. Since the slow onset of tetracaine for epidural anaesthesia was clinically unacceptable, the addition of lidocaine or mepivacaine provided a local anaesthetic solution which afforded a relatively rapid onset of action and prolonged duration of anaesthesia.

The introduction of bupivacaine and etidocaine provides the anaesthesiologist with anaesthetic solutions which possess a reasonably rapid onset of action and a prolonged duration. In addition, some studies have shown that a mixture of chloroprocaine and bupivacaine results in a duration of anaesthesia which is shorter than usually obtains when bupivacaine alone is employed. This decrease in duration has been attributed, in part, to the low pH of chloroprocaine solutions. Reduction in pH will decrease the amount of bupivacaine available in the uncharged base form, which may reduce the number of molecules able to penetrate the nerve sheath. Moreover, data from isolated nerve studies suggest that competition may exist between local anaesthetics for receptor sites in the nerve membrane. Occupation of receptor sites by chloroprocaine may decrease the number of binding sites for bupivacaine, which again would result in a decreased duration of action.

Another potential problem in terms of combining local anaesthetics concerns the systemic toxicity of such mixtures, since animal studies have indicated that the toxicity of local anaesthetics is additive.

In summary, there is little scientific basis for the use of mixtures of local anaesthetics for epidural blockade. Etidocaine and bupivacaine provide a clinically acceptable onset and duration of action. In addition, epidural catheter techniques can be employed for the initial administration of a rapid-acting agent such as chloroprocaine or lidocaine followed later by the administration of a long acting anaesthetic drug if desired.

Factors influencing epidural anaesthesia

The quality of epidural blockade will be influenced primarily by the local anaesthetic employed. The characteristics of the various agents have been presented above. Other factors that may influence the adequacy of epidural blockade include (a) dose, volume and concentration of the local anaesthetic agent, (b) addition of a vasoconstrictor to the local anaesthetic solution, (c) site and speed of injection, (d) patient position, and (e) patient age, height and clinical status.

Dose, volume and concentration of the local anaesthetic agent

The volume of the anaesthetic solution administered into the epidural space may influence the vertical spread of anaesthesia. For example, 30 ml of 1% lidocaine produced a level of analgesia following lumbar epidural administration which was 4.3 dermatomes higher than that achieved by 10 ml of 3% lidocaine. However, the relationship between spread and volume of anaesthetic solution is neither linear nor predictable. The essential qualities of epidural anaesthesia, that is, onset, depth and duration of sensory analgesia and motor blockade, are related to the mass of drug rather than to variations in volume or concentration of solution. For example, a comparison of 600 mg prilocaine administered epidurally either as 30 ml of a 2% solution or as 20 ml of a 3% solution failed to show any difference in onset, adequacy and duration of anaesthesia, and onset, depth and duration of motor blockade (Fig. 3:12). An increase in the dosage of local anaesthetic administered epidurally will tend to decrease the onset time, increase the frequency of satisfactory anaesthesia, and significantly prolong the duration of anaesthesia. Studies with bupivacaine administered epidurally in obstetrics have shown that increasing the concentration from 0.125% to 0.5% while maintaining the same volume of injection shortened the latency time, improved the incidence of satisfactory analgesia and increased the duration of sensory anaesthesia (Fig. 3:13). In addition, the degree and duration of motor blockade was also enhanced by an increase in the concentration and dosage of bupivacaine. Since the primary mechanism of epidural anaesthesia is believed to involve spinal root blockade, the main anaesthetic determinant should be the transdural drug gradient, which in turn is a function of the epidural drug mass, i.e. the product of volume times concentration.

Fig. 3:12 Relationship between volume and concentration of prilocaine and onset, duration and adequacy of analgesia and muscle relaxation.

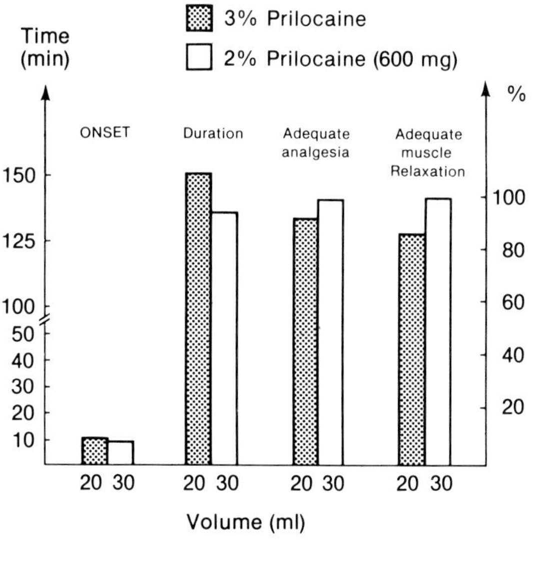

Addition of a vasoconstrictor to the local anaesthetic solution

Epinephrine is frequently added to local anaesthetic solutions intended for epidural administration. The anaesthetic properties of local anaesthetics are usually enhanced by the addition of epinephrine which increases the depth of blockade and significantly prolongs the duration of anaesthesia (Fig. 3:13). The effect of epinephrine is believed to be related primarily to its effect on the local vasculature, which causes a decrease in absorption of the local anaesthetic. Thus, more of the agent remains in the epidural space and is available for diffusion to the spinal roots and cord to produce a more profound degree and longer duration of anaesthesia. A 1:200,000 (5 µg. ml^{-1}) concentration of epinephrine is usually employed and has been demonstrated to be optimal when used in conjunction with lidocaine. While other vasoconstrictor agents such as phenylephrine have also been used as additives to solutions of local anaesthetics intended for epidural anaesthesia, the available evidence suggests that epinephrine is the most effective vasoconstrictor.

Fig. 3:13 Effect of epinephrine on onset, duration and frequency of complete analgesia of bupivacaine.

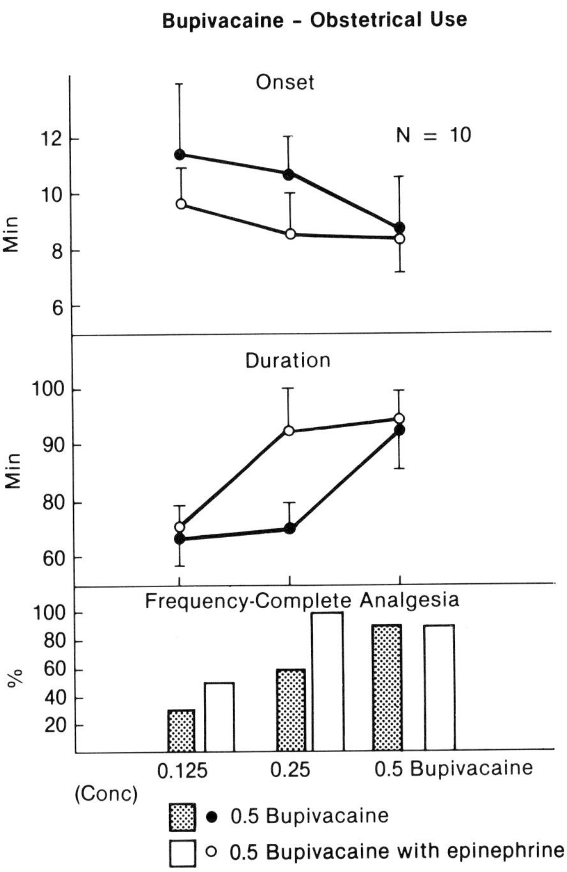

Prilocaine, bupivacaine and etidocaine administered epidurally do not appear to benefit as much as lidocaine from the addition of epinephrine. The decreased vasodilator action of prilocaine compared with lidocaine is believed to be responsible for the reduced effect of added epinephrine. In the case of bupivacaine and etidocaine, their high lipid solubility may be responsible for the diminished effect. These agents are taken up substantially by epidural fat and then slowly released, which contributes to their prolonged duration of action. Thus, the addition of epinephrine does not markedly prolong duration. The effect of epinephrine on the frequency and duration of adequate anaesthesia is dependent on the concentration of bupivacaine employed for epidural blockade. Concentrations of 0.125% to 0.5% of this agent have been used for epidural analgesia during labour, while 0.5% and 0.75% bupivacaine are most commonly employed for epidural anaesthesia in surgical patients. The frequency of adequate anaesthesia and the duration of sensory analgesia were markedly improved when epinephrine 1:200,000 was added to 0.25% bupivacaine for epidural blockade in obstetrical patients (Fig. 3:13). However, the addition of epinephrine to 0.5% and 0.75% bupivacaine was not associated with a significant improvement in the frequency of adequate anaesthesia. The duration was prolonged in some studies but not in others. Addition of epinephrine to either bupivacaine or etidocaine does appear to increase the degree of motor blockade.

Site and speed of injection

Because of variations in the diameter of the epidural space, injection of local anaesthetics into different sites will produce marked differences in the spread of anaesthesia. For example, injections of small volumes, i.e. 3-8 ml, into the relatively narrow midthoracic epidural space results in a discrete but wide segmental block (Fig. 3:14). Lumbar epidural administration requires the use of volumes of 10-25 ml to achieve surgical anaesthesia. Cephalad spread occurs more easily than caudad spread following lumbar epidural injections, due in part to the negative intrathoracic pressure and to the resistance afforded by the narrowing of the epidural space at the lumbar sacral junction. A significant delay and/or absence of analgesia at the first and second sacral segments is frequently observed following lumbar epidural injections. This has been attributed in part to the narrowing of the epidural space at the lumbosacral junction and also to the thickness of the spinal roots in this area. Caudal anaesthesia usually requires greater amounts of drug and little cephalad spread beyond the lumbosacral junction may occur because of the peculiar anatomy of the epidural space in this region.

Rate of injection appears to have little effect on the profile of epidural anaesthesia. Twenty millilitres of 2% lidocaine injected into the lumbar epidural space at a rate of 1 $ml.s^{-1}$ and 1 ml.3 s^{-1} did not influence the duration of anaesthesia or motor block or the level of anaesthesia in a significant manner. Of greater clinical importance, perhaps, is the greater patient discomfort which appears to be associated with the rapid injection of local anaesthetics into the epidural space, and the increased risk of serious toxicity if the drug is injected intravascularly.

Patient position

Posture was originally thought to influence the onset, spread and duration of epidural analgesia. However, studies involving the use of radio-opaque solutions and radio-isotopes administered into the epidural space failed to demonstrate any effect of posture on the spread of these materials in the epidural space. Controversy exists concerning the onset, spread and duration of sensory anaesthesia on the dependent and non-dependent side following epidural administration of local anaesthetics to patients in the lateral decubitus position. Several studies have shown a more rapid onset of analgesia and a higher dermatomal level on the dependent side. Other investigators have failed to confirm these findings. For example, a study involving patients scheduled for total hip replacements showed that maintenance of patients in a lateral position with the surgical side in a non-dependent position did not affect the maximum spread or duration of anaesthesia on the dependent and non-dependent sides. In general, patient position per se does not appear to predictably influence the spread or duration of epidural anaesthesia in a fashion similar to that following the administration of local anaesthetics into the subarachnoid space.

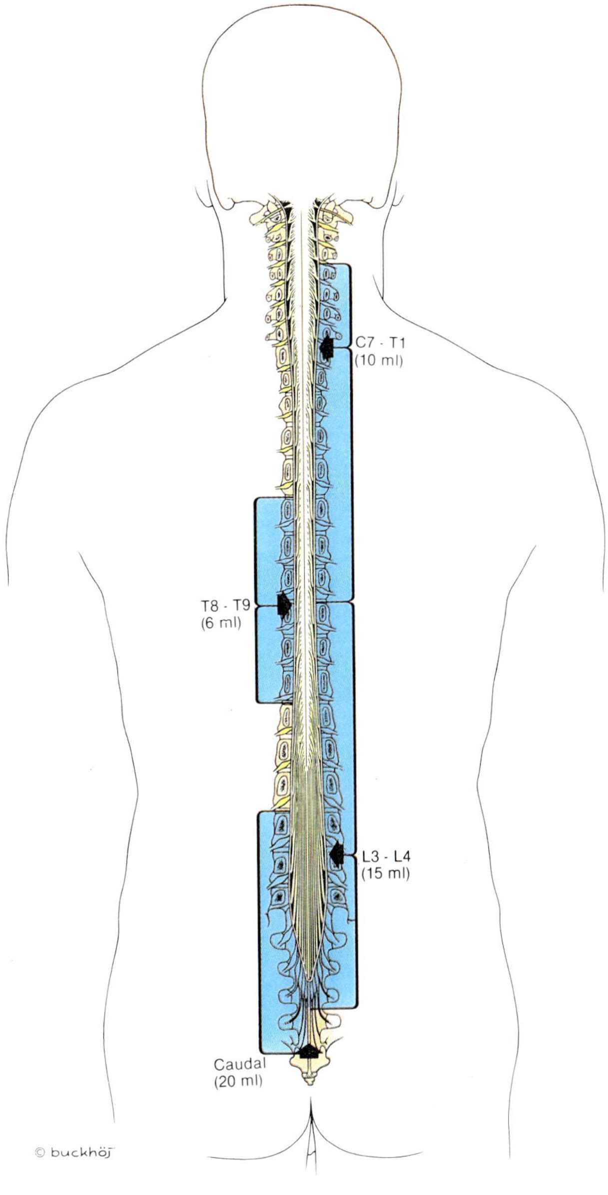

Fig. 3:14 Effect of the site of epidural administration on spread of a local anaesthetic solution.

Patient age, height, and physical status

Discrepancies exist between studies which have evaluated the influence of age and height of patients on the spread of anaesthetics in the epidural space. Originally the level of epidural block was reported to be related to height and age. Other investigators have failed to demonstrate any correlation between age, height and spread of radio-opaque material in the epidural space, and have concluded that the degree of vertical spread in the epidural space is dependent to a greater extent on the soft tissue content of the epidural space and that escape of solution via intravertebral foramina even in young people is of little significance. More recent studies comparing the spread of anaesthetic solution in patients of varying age have shown little correlation between the maximal dermatomal analgesic level obtained and the age of patients up to the age of 40 years. Patients 40 years and older did show a greater spread of epidural anaesthesia compared with patients less than 40 years of age when the volume and dose of local anaesthetic solution was the same in both groups. However, the mean difference between the various age groups was only 2-3 spinal segments.

Pregnancy is believed to affect the level of epidural anaesthesia. For example, similar levels of anaesthesia were obtained following the use of 6-10 ml of 2% lidocaine in obstetrical patients and 15-30 ml of 2% lidocaine in non-pregnant patients. This difference is believed to be related to inferior vena caval compression in pregnancy, which results in a marked distension of the epidural venous plexus. It is possible to mimic this situation in non-pregnant animals by placing an inflatable balloon in the inferior vena cava. Under these conditions an exaggerated rate of epidurally administered contrast media has been observed. The distended venous plexuses would occupy more space, thereby decreasing the diameter of the epidural cylinder and facilitating the vertical spread of epidurally administered anaesthetic solutions. However, almost full distension of veins occurs at a relatively low pressure (7-10 torr), and it is probable that, in the supine position, the venous plexus is fully dilated even in non-pregnant patients.

Recent studies suggest that the greater sensitivity and spread of epidural anaesthetics in pregnant patients may be related to hormonal rather than mechanical factors. The dose per segment requirement of epidurally administered local anaesthetics was decreased in patients during their first trimester of pregnancy compared with a similar group of non-pregnant patients. Since distension of epidural veins by inferior vena caval occlusion is not a factor at this early stage of pregnancy, the increased sensitivity to local anaesthetics is believed to be related to hormonal influences. Moreover, isolated nerve studies have confirmed a more rapid onset of conduction block in nerves from pregnant rabbits than in nerves from non-pregnant animals.

Opioids for epidural use

In recent years opioids such as morphine have been administered intrathecally or epidurally for the treatment of both acute postoperative pain and various chronic pain syndromes. The rationale for the use of epidural opioids was based on the discovery of specific opioid receptors in the spinal cord and the presence of naturally occurring opioid substances, enkephalins, which function as neurotransmitters at specific neurons in the spinal cord. The enkephalin neurons have been found to exist primarily in the substantia gelatinosa of the dorsal horn. As indicated previously, nociceptive fibres form a series of synapses in this region of the spinal cord. It is believed that the excitatory neurotransmitter, substance P, is probably released at nerve endings in the spinal cord and then activates postsynaptic neurons for transmission of nociceptive impulses to the brain (Fig. 3:15).

Enkephalin neurons impinge on the presynaptic terminals of the nociceptive fibres. Enkephalins, which are relatively small peptides, are released and interact with specific opioid receptors on the presynaptic nerve terminals to decrease the release of substance P. In this fashion the enkephalin system performs a modulating or inhibitory function in the transmission of nociceptive information.

Opioid receptors which modify the perception of pain are also located in various regions of the brain. Parenterally administered opioids act at these receptors to produce their analgesic effect. The discovery of opioid receptors in the spinal cord led to the intrathecal or epidural administration of various opioids in an attempt to activate the receptors in the substantia gelatinosa without influencing similar receptors in the brain. This resulted in the production of significant analgesia without nerve block, and the technique has been widely used for the treatment of both acute and chronic pain states.

Fig. 3:15 Diagram depicting substance P as the nociceptive transmitter agent in the spinal cord and the location of opioid receptors.

1. Large presynaptic fibre
2. Small presynaptic fibre
3. Opioid receptors
4. Substance P
5. Dorsal horn
6. Postsynaptic afferent fibre

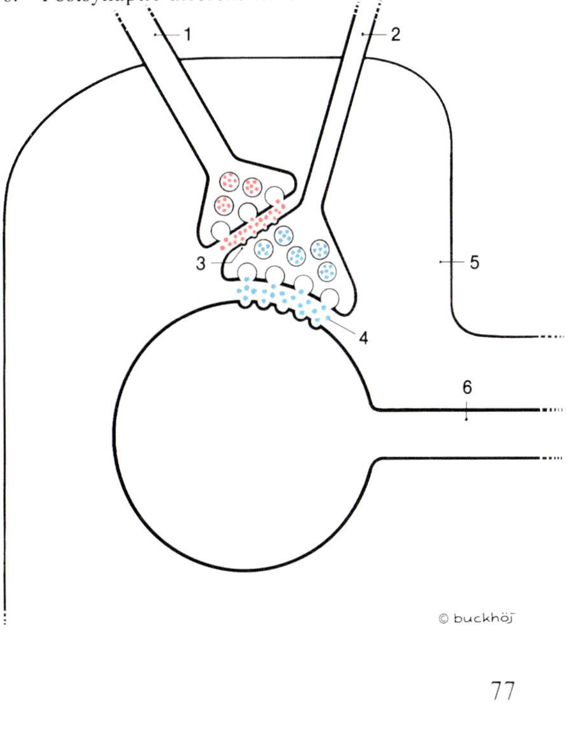

A comparison of the duration of analgesia following the intramuscular and epidural administration of morphine is indicative of the presence of opioid receptors in the spinal cord (Fig. 3:16). The absorption and blood levels of morphine following i.m. or epidural injections are similar. However, i.m. morphine produces a duration of analgesia of approximately 4 h, compared with a duration of 10-24 h following epidural administration.

All the narcotic analgesics are effective when administered epidurally. The primary difference between the various agents is related to their onset and duration of action and this appears to be a function of the lipid solubility of the different agents (Table 3:4).

Onset of analgesia

The onset of action of epidurally administered opioids varies widely between agents and appears to be related to their lipid solubility (Table 3:4). A comparison of the onset of analgesia in human volunteers following the epidural administration of morphine, hydromorphone and methadone revealed that morphine, which is the most hydrophilic agent, showed the longest average onset time – approximately 35 min. Methadone, which was the most lipophilic agent, produced signs of sensory analgesia after 17 min, while hydromorphone, which is intermediate in terms of its lipophilicity, had an average onset time of 23 min. Other studies have demonstrated that fentanyl, which is very lipophilic, usually induces sensory analgesia within 10 min following epidural administration. The differences in onset of action probably reflect the time required to diffuse from the epidural space across the dura mater into cerebrospinal fluid and ultimately into the spinal cord.

Fig. 3:16 Relationship between the plasma levels of epidurally and intramuscularly administered morphine and the duration of analgesia. (Modified from R. Watson.)

1. Epidural morphine plasma level
2. I.m. morphine plasma level
3. I.m. morphine analgesia
4. Epidural morphine analgesia

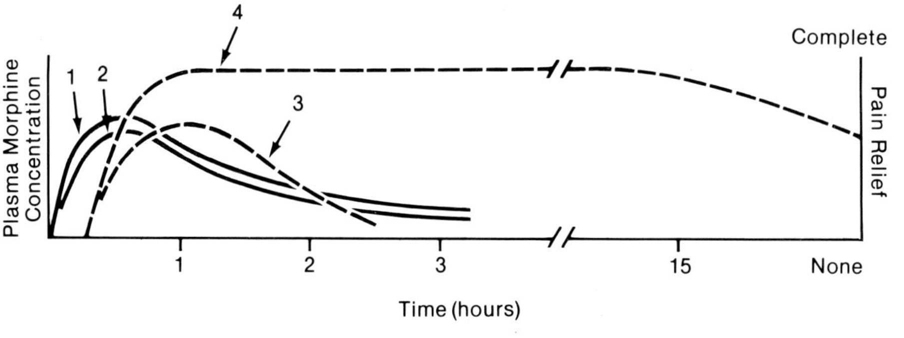

Duration of analgesia

Large variations in the duration of sensory analgesia have been reported following the epidural administration of opioids (Table 3:4). For example, 2-10 mg morphine injected into the epidural space produced sensory analgesic durations of 2-36 h. A general relationship exists between the degree of lipophilicity of the various agents and the average duration of sensory analgesia achieved. Epidural administration of methadone, hydromorphone and morphine in human volunteers resulted in average durations of sensory analgesia varying from 7 h for methadone, which is the most lipophilic, to 14 h for hydromorphone and 22 h for the least lipophilic agent, morphine. Other studies have reported durations of analgesia of 4-6 h for fentanyl and 6-8 h for pethidine, which are also more lipophilic than morphine. Thus, while the more lipid-soluble agents can penetrate the dura mater more rapidly, their high lipid solubility also allows for a more rapid diffusion away from the spinal cord and subarachnoid space, resulting in a shorter duration of action.

Table 3:4
Epidural Narcotics
Relationship of Lipid Solubility to Onset and Duration of Analgesia

Drug	Partition Coefficient	Onset Time (min)	Duration (hours)
Morphine	0.79	15-60	5-36
Pethidine	2.72	5-15	4-18
Methadone	3.93	10-20	6-8
Fentanyl	4.05	5-10	4

Dosage of epidural opioids

The optimal dosage of epidural opioids required for maximal analgesic activity without severe side effects varies widely as a function of the agent employed, patient status and concomitant use of epinephrine.

Doses of morphine varying from 2 to 20 mg have been employed for epidural use. Several dose-response studies have been conducted which suggest that the optimal dose of morphine for sensory analgesia following epidural administration is 5-10 mg for the relief of acute postoperative pain (Fig. 3:17). The original belief that very small doses were effective has proved to be unfounded. In obstetrics, the use of morphine has proven disappointing in terms of adequate control of pain during labour. A great variation exists in the doses of epidural morphine which have been used for the treatment of chronic pain patients. Doses of 2-20 mg morphine have been administered epidurally for chronic pain management with varying degrees of success.

Fig. 3:17 Dose-response relationship between degree of pain and the dose of epidurally administered morphine.

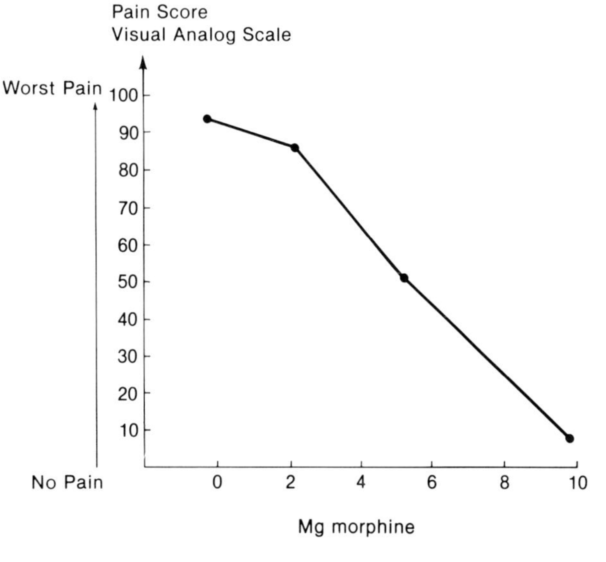

Adequate dose-response studies have not been well conducted with other opioid analgesics. In general, doses of 50-100 μg fentanyl, 50-100 mg pethidine and 1 mg methadone and hydromorphone (i.e., similar to the doses used for intramuscular use) have been administered epidurally for relief of acute postoperative pain.

Epinephrine has been added to certain opioids in an attempt to produce a more profound and prolonged state of analgesia. Epinephrine was reported to prolong the duration of sensory analgesia produced by epidural morphine and increase the adequacy of pain relief provided by pethidine. The action of epinephrine is presumed to be related to its vasoconstrictor properties which would decrease the rate of vascular absorption of the opioid analgesics similar to its effect with local anaesthetics. On the other hand, some evidence suggests that adrenergic receptors may be present in the spinal cord which can modulate the transmission of nociceptive impulses and these may be activated by epinephrine.

A comparison of the analgesic effects of bupivacaine and morphine administered epidurally for the treatment of acute postoperative pain has been carried out. Bupivacaine was found to produce an average duration of sensory analgesia of approximately 5 h while 10 mg morphine was associated with an average duration of sensory analgesia of 15 h. Moreover, while only 20% of the patients in the bupivacaine group had analgesia lasting longer than 6 h, all the patients in the morphine group were analgesic for longer than 6 h. However, the onset of analgesia produced by morphine was relatively slow compared with the time of onset following bupivacaine. Thus, some investigators have advocated the combined use of local anaesthetics with narcotic analgesics for control of postoperative pain in order to obtain both a rapid onset and a prolonged duration of analgesia.

References & Bibliography

Behar, M. and Magora, F. (1979). Epidural morphine in treatment of pain. The Lancet 1:527.

Blaustein, M.P. and Goldman, D.E. (1966). Action of anionic and cationic nerve-blocking agents: experiment and interpretation. Science 153:429.

Bridenbaugh, P.O., Tucker, G.T., Moore, D.C., Bridenbaugh, L.D., Thompson, G.E. and Balfour, R.I. (1974). Role of epinephrine in regional block anesthesia with etidocaine: a double-blind study. Anesth. Analg. 53:430.

Bromage, P.R. (1980). Epidural narcotics in volunteers: sensitivity to pain and to carbon dioxide. Pain 9:145.

Bromage, P.R. (1980): Epidural narcotics for postoperative analgesia. Anesth. Analg. 59:473.

Bromage, P.R. (1962). Exaggerated spread of epidural analgesia in arteriosclerotic patients. Dosage in relation to biological and chronological aging. Brit. Med. J. 2:1634.

Bromage, P.R. (1975). Mechanism of action of extradural analgesia. Brit. J. Anaesth. 47:199.

Bromage, P.R. (1982). Rostral spread of epidural morphine. Anesthesiology 56:431.

Bromage, P.R. (1962). Spread of analgesic solutions in the epidural space and their site of action: a statistical study. Brit. J. Anaesth. 34:161.

Buckley, F.P., Littlewood, D.G., Covino, B.G. and Scott, D.B. (1978). Effects of adrenaline and the concentration of solution on extradural block with etidocaine. Brit. J. Anaesth. 50:171.

Corke, B.C., Carlson, C.G. and Dettbarn, W. (1984). The influence of 2-chloroprocaine on the subsequent analgesic potency of bupivacaine. Anesthesiology 60:25.

Covino, B.G. and Vassallo, H.G. (1976). Local Anesthetics. Mechanisms of action and clinical use. New York, Grune & Stratton.

Covino, B.G. (1983): Pharmacology of local anesthetic agents. Seminars in Anesthesia 2:10.

Crawford, O.B. (1964). Comparative evaluation in peridural anesthesia of lidocaine, mepivacaine and L 67, a new local anesthetic agent. Anesthesiology 25:321.

Datta, S., Lambert, D.H., Gregus, J., Gissen, A.J. and Covino, B.G. (1983). Differential sensitivities of mammalian nerve fibers during pregnancy. Anesth. Analg. 62:1070.

deJong, R.H. (ed.) (1977). Local Anesthetics. 2nd Edition, Springfield, Charles C. Thomas.

Erdemir, H.A., Soper, L.E. and Sweet, R.B. (1965). Studies of factors affecting peridural anesthesia. Anesth. Analg. 44:400.

Fagraeus, L., Urban, B.J. and Bromage, P.R. (1983). Spread of epidural analgesia in early pregnancy. Anesthesiology 58:184.

Hartrick, C.T., Raj, P.P., Direkes, W.E., Jr. and Denson, D.D. (1984). Compounding of bupivacaine and mepivacaine for regional anesthesia. A safe practice? Reg. Anesth. 9:94.

Henre, F.W., Moyes, A.Z., Senfield, R.M. and Lilly, E.J. (1965). Continuous lumbar peridural anesthesia in obstetrics, II. Use of minimal amounts of local anesthetics during labor. Anesth. Analg. 44:89.

Littlewood, D.G., Buckley, P., Covino, B.G., Scott, D.B. and Wilson, J. (1979). Comparative study of various local anaesthetic solutions in block in labour. Brit. J. Anaesth. 51:47S.

Martin, R. (1982). Epidural morphine for postoperative pain relief: a doseresponse curve. Anesthesiology 56:423.

Modig, J. and Paalzow, L. (1981). A comparison of epidural morphine and epidural bupivacaine for postoperative pain relief. Acta Anaesth. Scand. 25:437.

Nordberg, G. and Hedner, T. (1983). Pharmacokinetic aspects of epidural morphine analgesia. Anesthesiology 58:545,

Park, W.Y., Hagins, F.M. and MacNamara, T.E. (1983). Lateral position and epidural anesthetic spread. Anesth. Analg. 62:245.

Park, W.Y., Massengale, M., Kim, S., Kwok, C.P. and MacNamara, T.E. (1980). Age and the spread of local anesthetic solutions in the epidural space. Anesth. Analg. 59:768.

Ritchie, J.M. and Ritchie, B.R. (1968). Local anesthetics: effect of pH on activity. Science 162:1394.

Ritchie, J.M., Ritchie, B. and Greengard, P. (1965). The active structure of local anesthetics. J. Pharmacol. Exp. Ther. 150:152.

Ritchie, J.M. (1975). Mechanism of action of local anaesthetic agents and biotoxins. Brit. J. Anaesth. 47:191.

Sayig, J.M. and Hehre, F.W. (1959). Effect of epinephrine on onset of anesthetic action of lidocaine in the peridural space in man. Anesth. Analg. 38:438.

Scott, D.B., McClure, J.H., Giasi, R.M., Seo, J. and Covino, B.G. (1980). Effects of concentration of local anaesthetic drugs in extradural block. Brit. J. Anaesth. 52:1033.

Seow, L.T., Lips, F.J. and Cousins, M.J. (1983). Effect of lateral posture on epidural blockade for surgery. Anaesth. Intens. Care 11:97.

Seow, L.T., Lips, F.J. Cousins, M.J. and Mather, L.W. (1982). Lidocaine and bupivacaine mixtures for epidural blockade. Anesthesiology 56:177.

Sharrock, N.E. (1978). Epidural anesthetic dose responses in patients 20 to 80 years old. Anesthesiology 49:425.

Sharrock, N.E. (1977). Lack of exaggerated spread of epidural anesthesia in patients with arteriosclerosis. Anesthesiology 47:307.

Strichartz, G. (1976). Molecular mechanisms of nerve block by local anesthetics. Anesthesiology 45:421

Yaksh, T.L. (1981). Spinal opiate analgesia: characteristics and principles of action. Pain 11:293.

Youngstrom, P.C. (1982). Pain relief and plasma concentrations from epidural and intramuscular morphine in post-cesarean patients. Anesthesiology 57:404.

4. Technical considerations

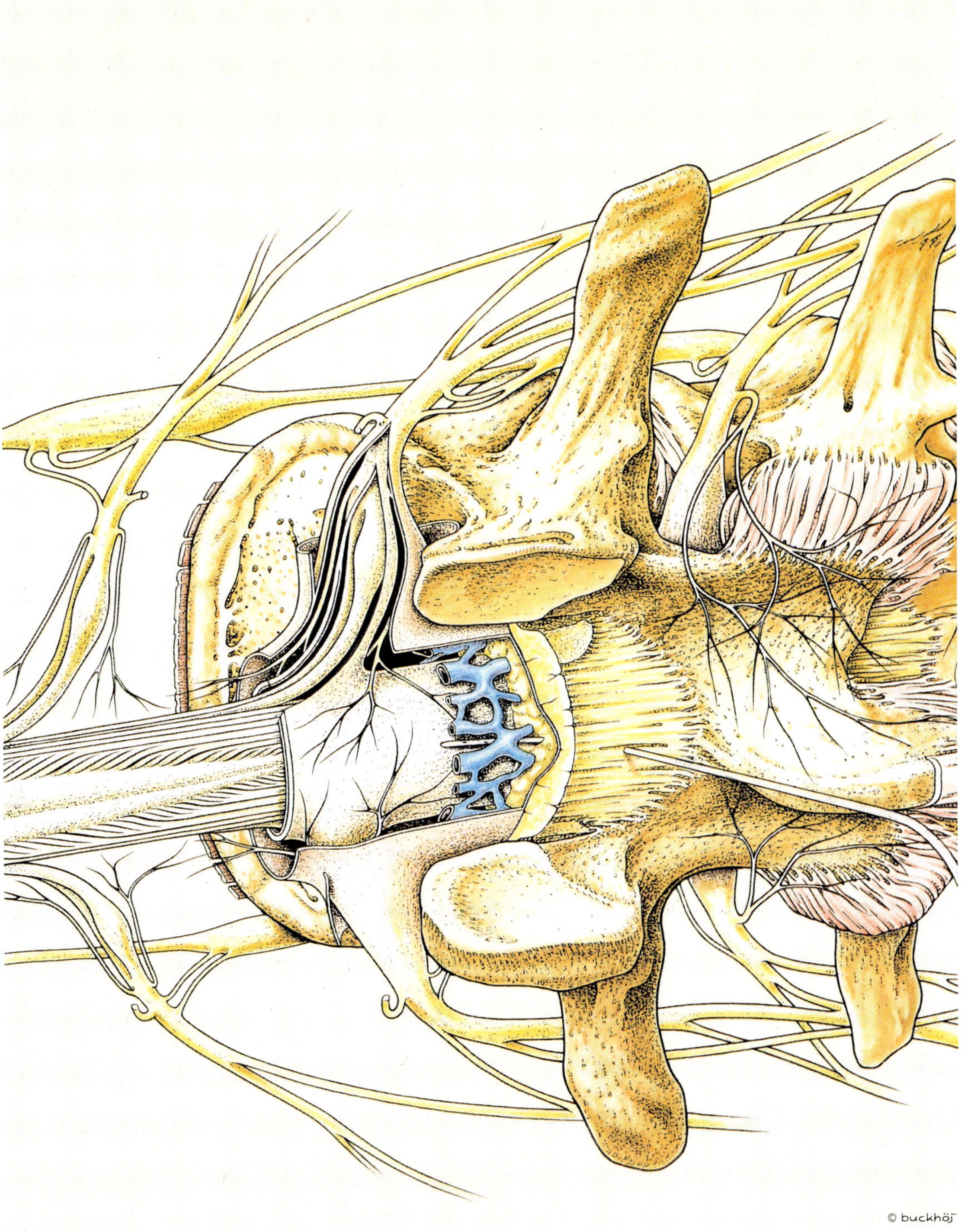

Anatomical landmarks

The most important bony landmarks for performance of epidural blockade are:

1. Vertebral spinal processes
2. Iliac crests
3. 12th ribs
4. Scapulae

The spinous processes clearly define the midline (Fig. 4:1). Sagging of the soft tissues, especially in obese patients, can be misleading, as the apparent midline may be several centimetres from the true midline. The identification of the individual lumbar vertebrae can be made by reference to the iliac crests, which are on a level with the fourth lumbar vertebra. Thus the interspinous space below is that between L_4 and L_5 (Fig. 4:1).

A line joining the tips of the 12th ribs is at the level of the L_2 spinous process.

The inferior angle of the scapula is at the level of T_7. A line joining the inferior aspect of the acromion is at the level of the T_2-T_3 interspace. The posterior superior iliac spines are at the level of the third sacral vertebra. In very obese patients it may be impossible to palpate the spinous processes and they must then be located with the epidural needle.

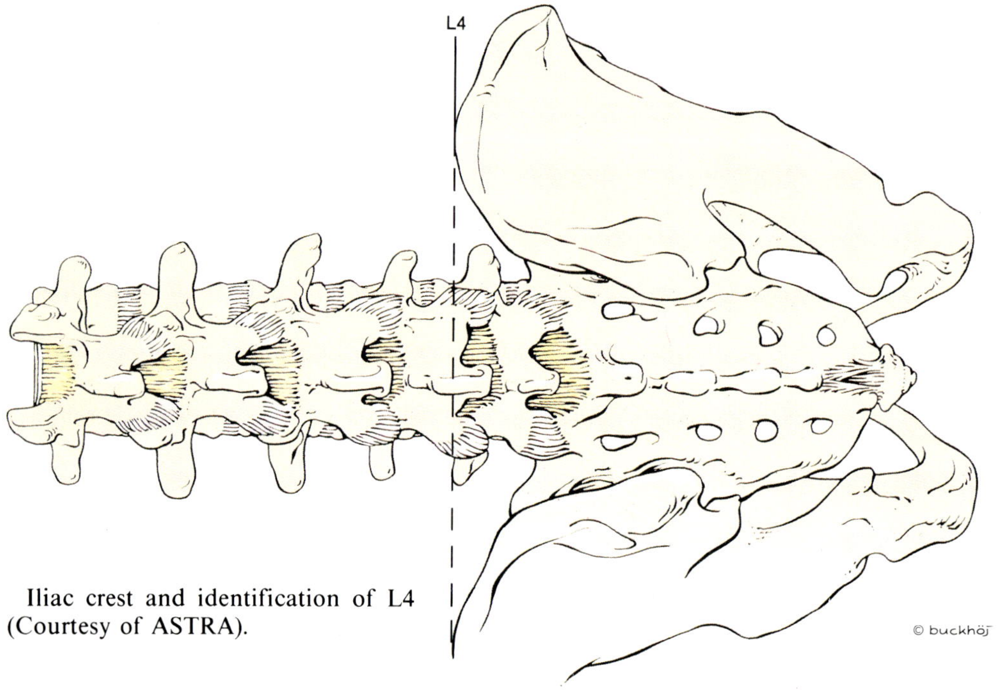

Fig. 4:1 Iliac crest and identification of L4 vertebra. (Courtesy of ASTRA).

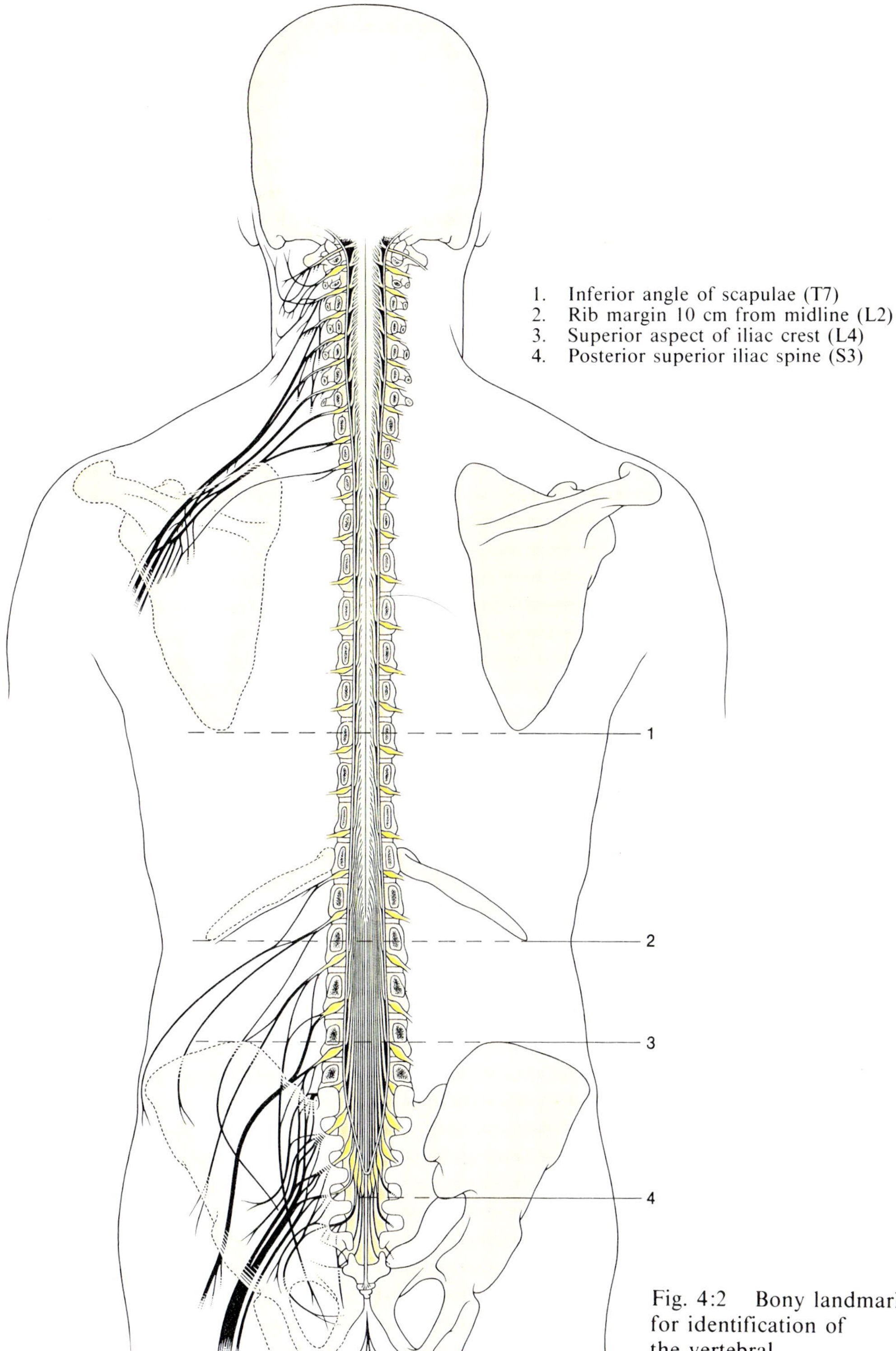

Fig. 4:2 Bony landmarks for identification of the vertebral spinous processes.

Lumbar epidural block

The epidural space is most easily entered in the lumbar region. Here the spinous processes are not angulated in relation to the vertebral body and the gap between adjacent laminae, covered by the ligamentum flavum, is wide. Moreover the spinal cord, which ends at the level of L_1, is not vulnerable to trauma from the needle.

Patient position

The patient must be positioned with the lumbar spine in maximal flexion so that the intervertebral spaces are opened out (Fig. 4:3a and b). This can be done in the lateral or the sitting position. For the former the patient is asked to raise the knees as high as possible in front of the abdomen and to lower the head towards the knees (Fig. 4:4a). In the sitting position the patient should be provided with a stool to put the feet on and instructed to lean forward with the elbows resting on the knees or on armrests (Fig. 4:4b).

Fig. 4:3 Radiograph of the lumbar spine in a. extension and b. flexion.

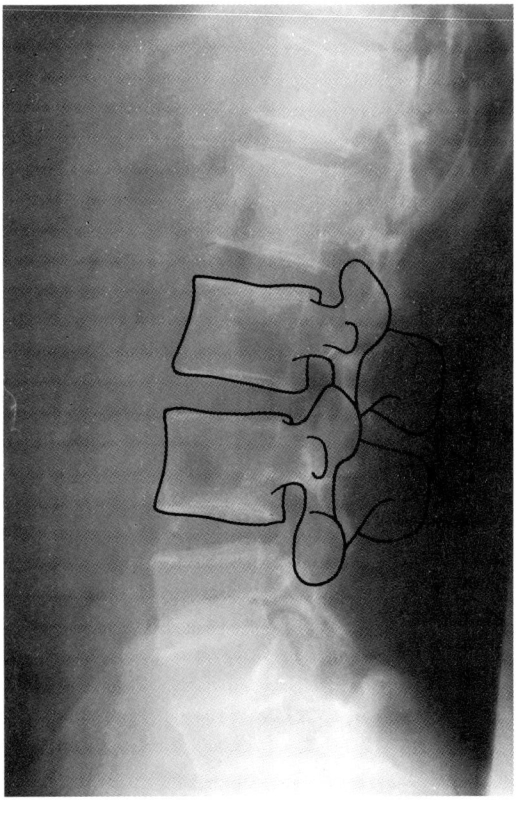

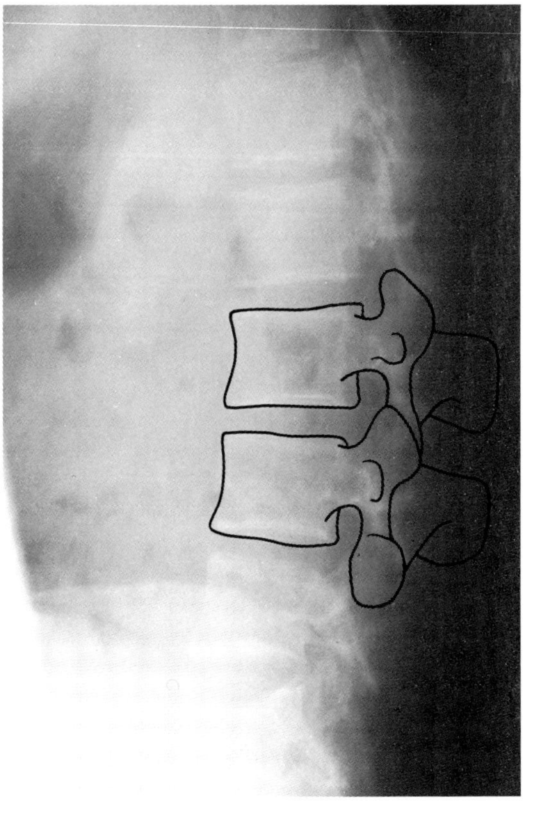

Equipment

Epidural pack

The instruments included in the sterile epidural pack will depend upon the personal preference of the anaesthetist. The most important item is the needle to be used in locating the epidural space (Fig. 4:5). That most commonly used is the Tuohy needle (Fig. 4:6), which is usually between 16 and 18 gauge. Its curved Huber point is designed to decrease the possibility of accidental puncture of the dura mater. In addition it facilitates the passage of a plastic catheter into the epidural space.

Some authorities like a rounded blunt needle end while others prefer a sharper point. The former is less likely to puncture the dura but requires more force to be pushed through the ligamentum flavum. The latter penetrates the ligament with less force, and care must be taken at the moment of entry into the epidural space.

Fig. 4:4 Patient position a. Lying horizontal b. Sitting upright. (Courtesy of ASTRA).

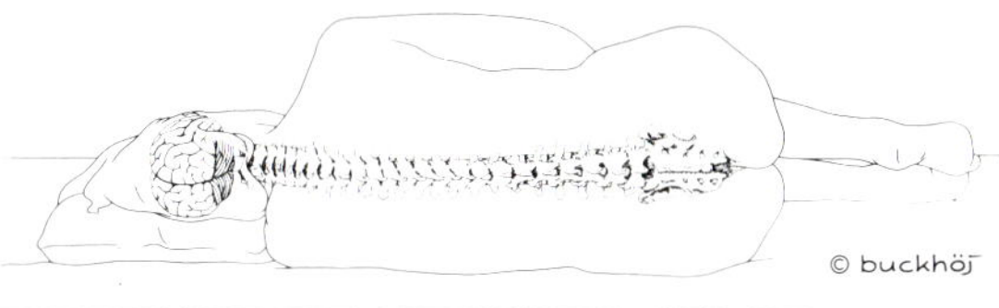

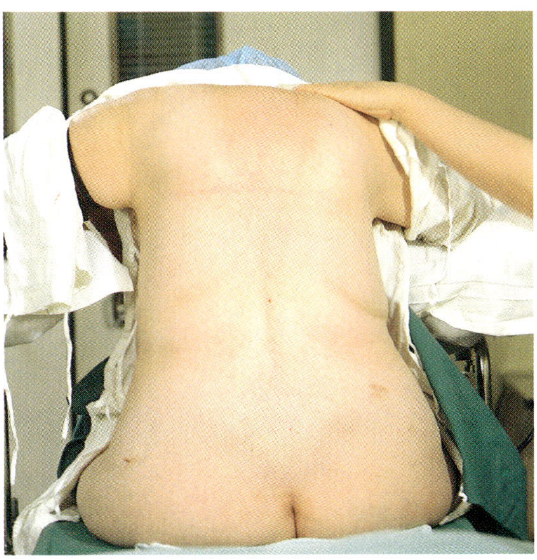

Fig. 4:5 Needles commonly used for epidural block A. Weiss needle (note wings and blunt point). B. Standard Tuohy needle (with sharper point). C. Crawford needle (note short bevel).

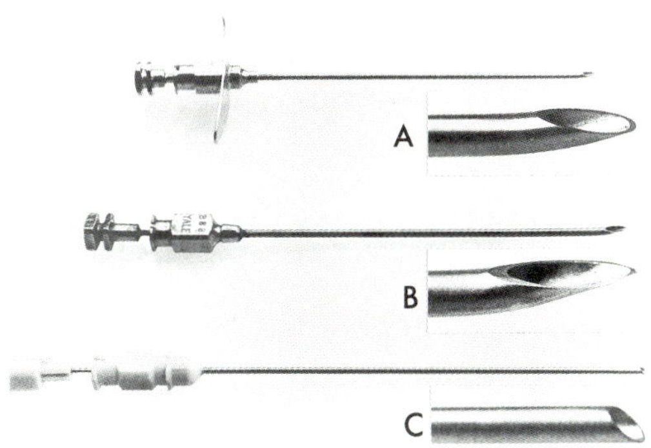

A modification of this needle, in which the shaft protrudes from the hub (Fig. 4:7), has advantages when any obstruction is met to the forward movement of the catheter.

A winged needle (Fig. 4:5) can be used and it allows both hands to grasp the needle during insertion into the epidural space. An alternative to the Tuohy needle is a Crawford needle (Fig. 4:5) which is a simple short bevelled straight needle, which is preferred by some for thoracic epidural block.

The epidural pack must also include

- Syringes. Again a personal choice. The recently introduced low resistance plastic syringes have advantages.

- Aspiration needles and intradermal needles.

- Ampoules or vials of local anaesthetic and normal saline.

- A stylet for making a hole in the skin prior to insertion of the Tuohy needle.

- Swabs, lotion pots and sterile drapes for cleaning the skin and draping the patient.

In addition a plastic catheter and possibly a bacterial filter should be available, either within the pack or in separate sterile packets.

Figs. 4:6 a. and b. Tuohy needle, showing different types of Huber point.

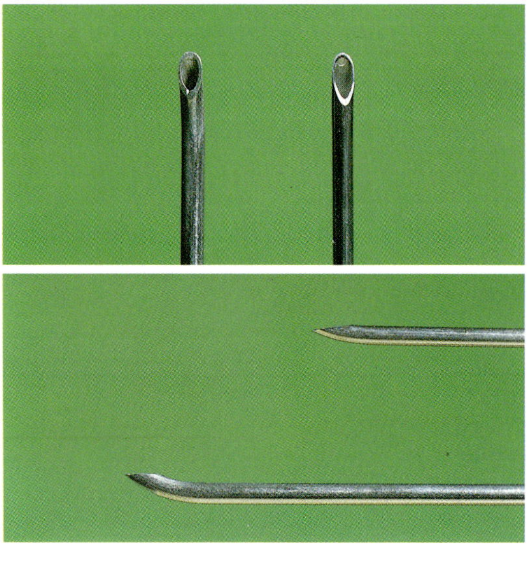

Fig. 4:7 Modified hub of Tuohy needle (Scott epidural needle).

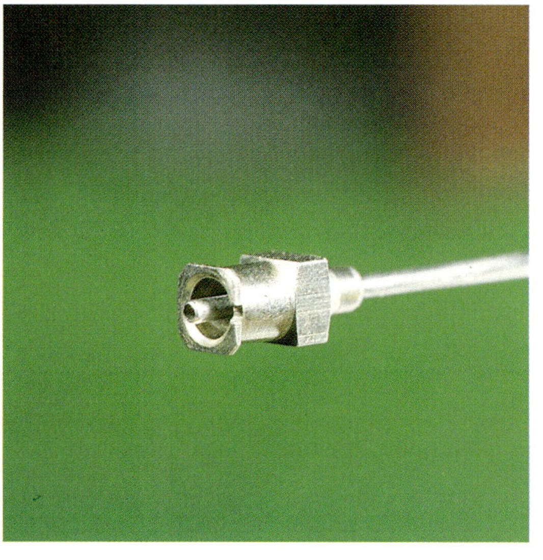

Procedure – Midline approach

Epidural blocks should only be performed where full anaesthetic facilities are available. A standard anaesthetic machine and all resuscitative equipment and drugs must be at hand.

An intravenous infusion should be set up as the first step. Blood pressure and heart rate should be recorded and many would insist that the electrocardiogram be displayed. The patient should be positioned as described above.

The bony landmarks are palpated. The iliac crest is felt at the level of the L_4 vertebra.

The L_1-L_2, L_3-L_4, and L_4-L_5 interspaces are those most commonly used.

All necessary sterile precautions must be taken. The equipment must of course be sterile. The anaesthetist should, at the minimum, don sterile rubber gloves, and some would insist on full gowning as well. The patient's back is prepared with an appropriate antiseptic solution as for a surgical operation, and sterile drapes applied.

An intradermal wheal is raised with local anaesthetic exactly over the chosen interspace. Subcutaneous infiltration may also be used.

A large sharp needle or a stylet is then pushed through the skin to allow easy penetration with the epidural needle.

Holding the skin firmly over the spinous process with the index and middle fingers of one hand, the epidural needle is inserted in the middle of the interspace at right angles to the skin. The skin should not be allowed to move, otherwise the needle may be inserted too far laterally.

The needle is advanced until it is firmly engaged in the interspinous ligament. It now has to penetrate the ligamentum flavum to reach the epidural space (Fig. 4:8). The stylet is withdrawn.

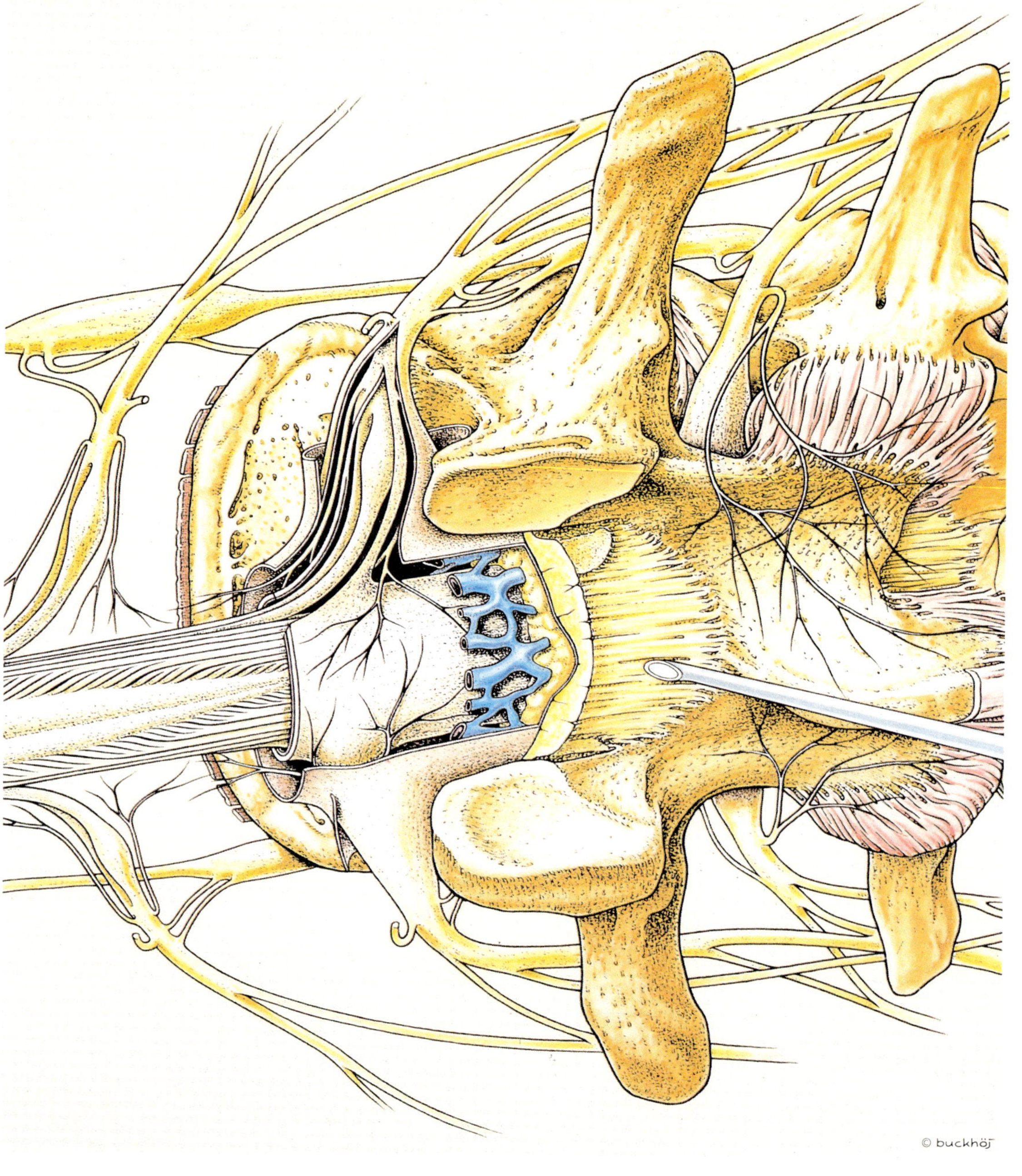

Fig. 4:8 Position of needle before penetration of ligamentum flavum.

Identification of the epidural space

Loss of resistance technique

The commonest method used is the loss of resistance technique. There are many variations of this technique, some using the hands and others with mechanical aids.

A syringe containing saline or air is attached to the needle lying in the interspinous ligament. Injection will be found to be difficult or impossible. The most difficult part of the technique to learn is the control of the advancing needle, which must not penetrate the epidural space beyond the needle bevel. The position of the hands and fingers on the needle and syringe are critical.

The index finger of the non-injecting hand may be held firmly against the patient's back to act as a resistance to sudden forward movement. The thumb and middle finger hold the needle hub (Fig. 4:9).

Alternatively the dorsum on the non-injecting hand is placed on the patient's back and the fingers can be turned back to hold the needle at its hub. The hand thus acts as an "opponens" to the advancing syringe and needle (Fig. 4:10).

This may even be exaggerated so that the hand grasps the lower end of the syringe (Fig. 4:11).

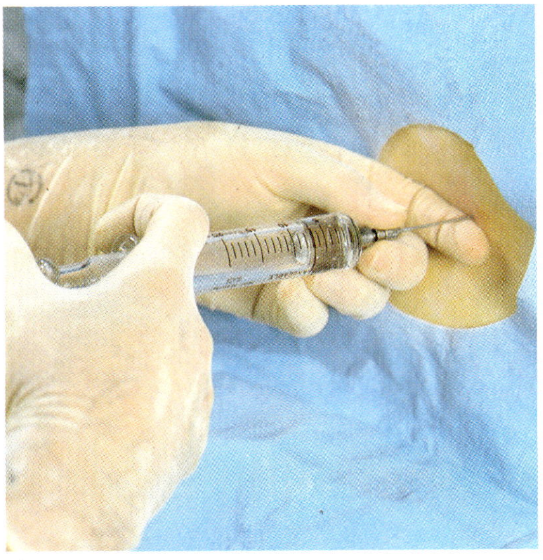

Fig. 4:9

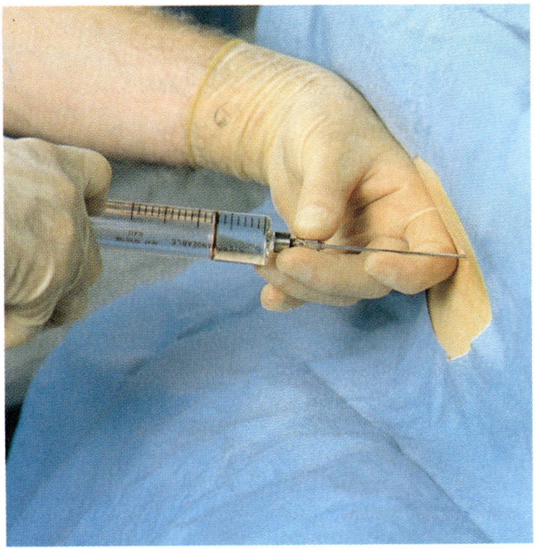

Fig. 4:10

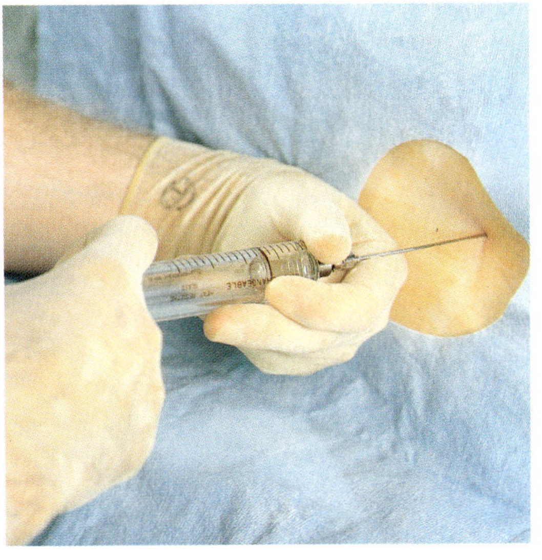

Fig. 4:11

Where advancement of the needle is relatively easy, continuous pressure on the syringe plunger can be used, care being taken that the needle is pushed through the ligamentum flavum slowly and without a sudden forward movement, which could lead to penetration of the dura mater.

As the needle is advanced, pressure is maintained on the plunger, noting the increased resistance of the ligamentum flavum. At the moment of entering thc cpidural space, saline or air can be injected with great ease.

The flow of fluid (or air) from the syringe as the needle enters the epidural space pushes the dura away from the needle point (Fig. 4:12a and b).

Figs. 4:12 Needle position a. Before and b. After penetration of the ligamentum flavum. Note that injection becomes easy when the ligament is passed and the injected fluid pushes the dura away from the needle.

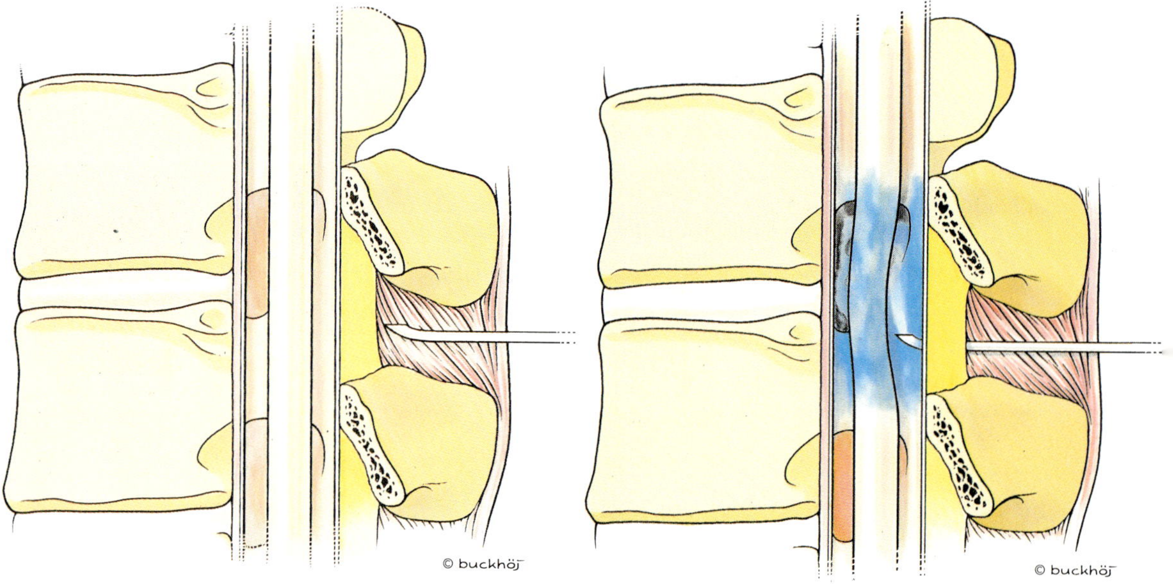

When a blunter needle is preferred or the ligaments are difficult to penetrate, then an intermittent technique can be used. Both hands push on the needle in a controlled way and the resistance to injection is tested after every millimetre of advancement (Fig. 4:13).

Mechanical aids include the Macintosh balloon, an intravenous infusion and a spring-loaded (Evans) syringe (Fig. 4:14). These allow two-handed advancement of the needle (which is helped by a winged needle) and the immediate identification of the epidural space as the resistance to injection disappears.

"Hanging drop" technique

The negative pressure that is often found within the epidural space is the basis for the "hanging-drop" technique. A winged needle is usually used and is advanced with both hands. A drop of fluid is placed at the end of the needle after engaging the interspinous ligament (Fig. 4:15). When the ligamentum flavum is penetrated the drop of fluid is sucked into the epidural space, and correct identification of the space can be confirmed by injection of fluid or air without resistance. Unfortunately a negative pressure cannot always be demonstrated and many anaesthetists feel this method is less reliable than the loss of resistance technique.

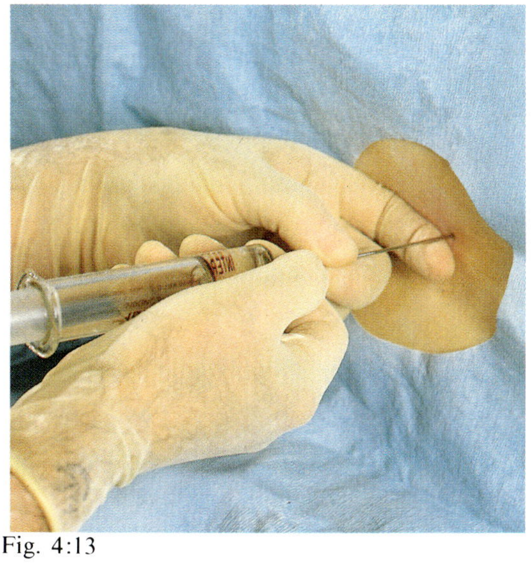

Fig. 4:13

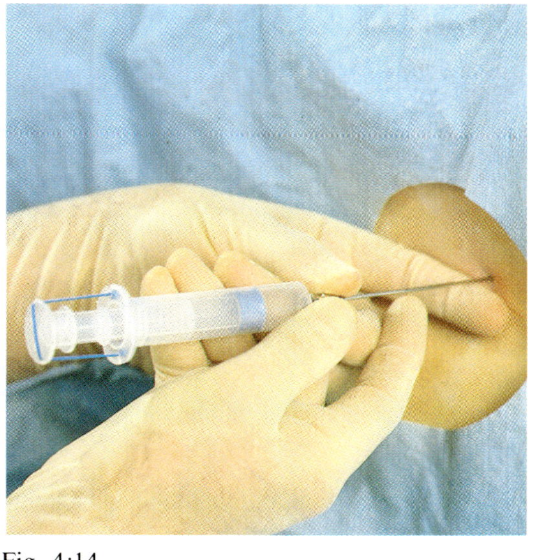

Fig. 4:14

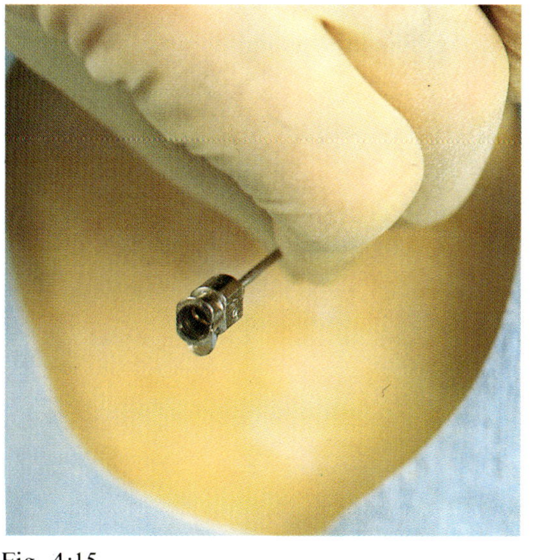

Fig. 4:15

Lateral or paramedian approach

Most anaesthetists prefer to use the midline approach particularly in the lumbar and lower thoracic region. Some, however, maintain that a slightly lateral insertion is easier. While this may be true in the mid-thoracic region, where the spinous processes are acutely angled, it does not apply at other sites where the spinous processes are horizontal or nearly so. It will be described briefly here but a more detailed account of its use in thoracic epidural block is given on page 100.

The needle is inserted about 1 - 1.5 cm lateral to the midline and on a level with the upper border of the spinous process below the chosen interspace. Thus the needle is not only more lateral but also inferior to the midline insertion (Fig. 4:16). It is aimed both upwards and inwards to penetrate the ligamentum flavum in the midline and should not therefore contact the spinous process. If bone is contacted, it will be the lamina of the vertebra, and the needle must be redirected so that it enters and penetrates the ligamentum flavum. Detection of the epidural space is as described above.

Catheter technique

If a prolonged nerve block is required, a plastic catheter can be introduced through the needle so that repeated injections can be made to provide a continuous epidural block for the duration of surgery and, if required, into the postoperative period. This, of course, also applies to epidural block used for relief of pain in labour.

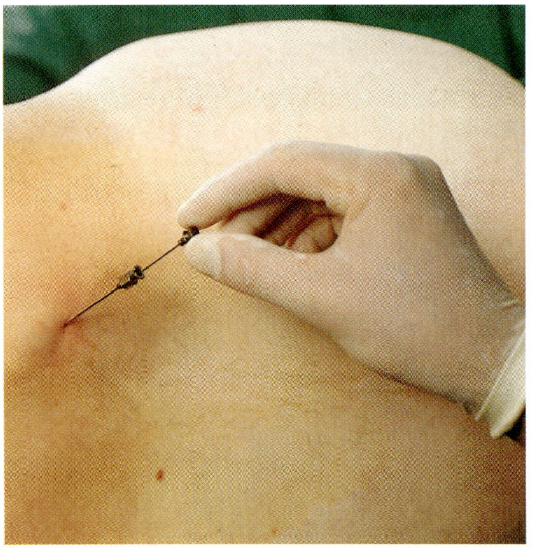

Fig. 4:16 Lateral or paramedian approach. The needle is inserted 1-1.5 cm lateral to the midline at the level of the upper border of the spinous process below the chosen vertebral interspace.

A plastic catheter with appropriate (5 cm) distance markings is used. It is passed through the needle and into the epidural space.

The catheter is rolled in one hand to prevent it falling into an unsterile area.

A slight resistance is felt as the catheter passes through the tip of the needle, when the second distance mark will just be visible at the hub (Fig. 4:17).

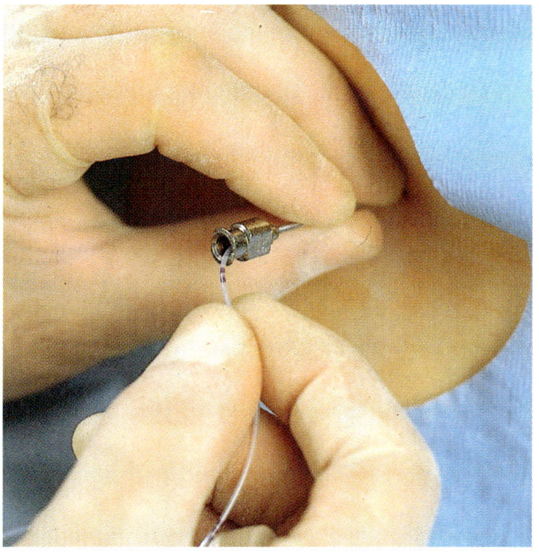

Fig. 4:17

By turning the needle, the Huber point can be directed cephalad or caudad. The catheter can therefore be advanced in either direction.

About 5 cm of catheter is advanced into the epidural space, when the third distance mark will be at or near the needle hub (Fig. 4:18).

The needle is then withdrawn carefully without removing the catheter, which is gently pushed forwards as the needle is being retracted.

The needle is completely removed from the patient (Fig. 4:19).

There are several different designs of catheter available. Some have a single terminal opening, while others have up to 3 lateral holes. Some are supplied with a stylet. Most are somewhat rigid at their tip, though a recently introduced catheter (Racz catheter) employs a stainless steel coil to make the tip very flexible, with less chance of penetrating the wall of an epidural vein. All are provided with a means of connecting the proximal end of the catheter to a syringe.

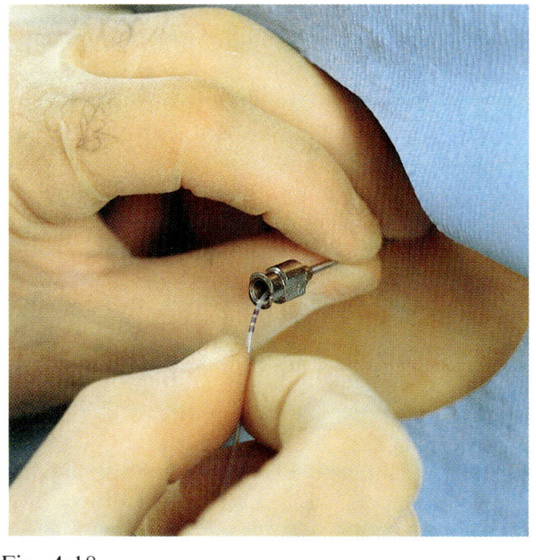

Fig. 4:18

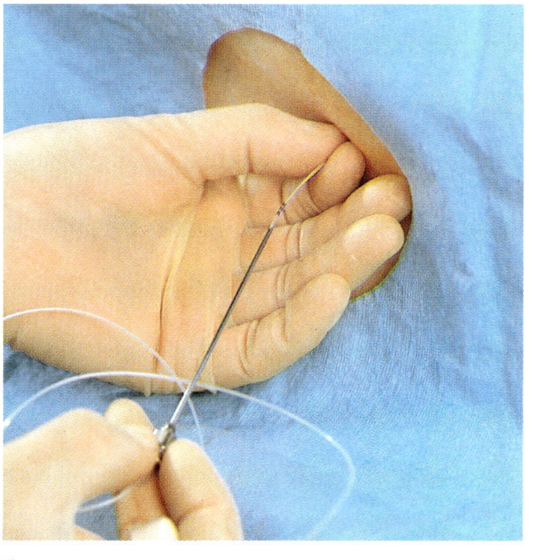

Fig. 4:19

A bacterial filter can be attached to the free end so that all fluid injected down the catheter is sterile.

Water-resistant strapping is used to keep the catheter in place (Fig. 4:20).

All injections can now be made near the patient's head (Fig. 4:21).

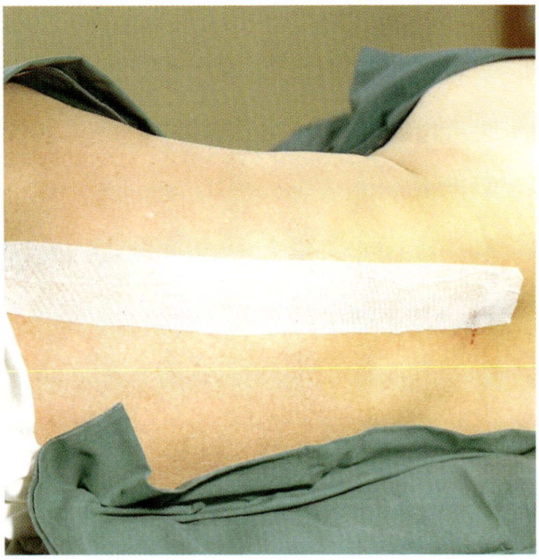

Fig. 4:20

Misplacement of needle or catheter

The anaesthetist must ensure that the needle tip or the catheter is in the epidural space. If the catheter has been incorrectly inserted and does not lie within the spinal canal, then no nerve block will result from the injection of local anaesthetic. This possibility must be entertained if there is no evidence of a nerve block within 15 20 min. The most likely position of the catheter in such a case is the sacrospinalis muscle, lateral to the spinous process. This can occur particularly in obese patients. The anaesthetist can be misled by the ease of injection, since a loss of resistance can occur when the needle deviates laterally from the interspinous ligament and reaches the muscular compartment.

In terms of patient safety, the anaesthetist must be able to diagnose both dural tap and inadvertent intravenous placement of the needle or catheter.

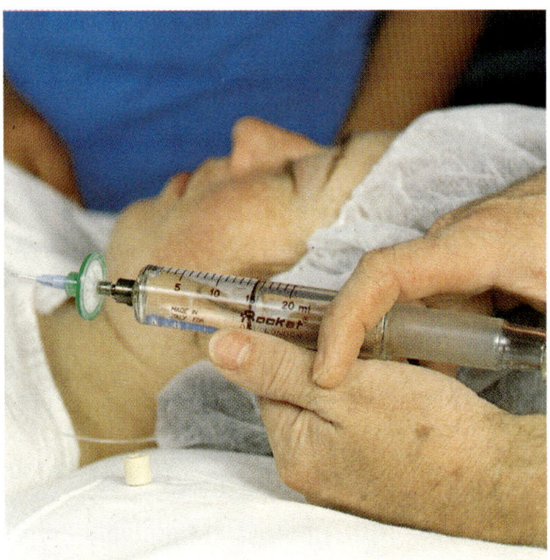

Fig. 4:21

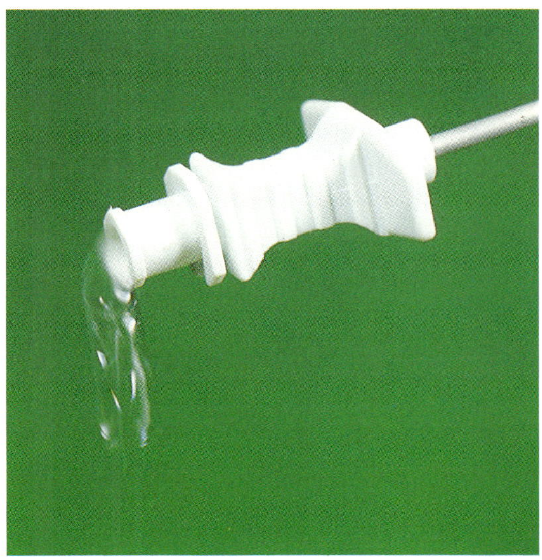

Fig. 4:22

Dural tap

Most dural taps are due to an uncontrolled sudden forward movement of the needle as the ligamentum flavum is penetrated. Dural tap will be diagnosed by removing the syringe and observing cerebrospinal fluid (CSF) escaping from the needle (Fig. 4:22). CSF may be distinguished from the fluid used in the syringe by its temperature or by the presence of glucose. If the subarachnoid space has been entered, the escape of CSF through the large bore needle is usually so copious that there is little doubt as to the true position of the needle.

Intravenous placement

Penetration of an epidural vein by the needle is easy to detect as blood flows freely from the needle hub. In such a case the needle must be withdrawn and the procedure repeated at the same or an adjacent vertebral interspace.

Intravascular placement of a catheter, however, may be much more difficult to diagnose. Catheters advanced through the needle can penetrate vein walls (Fig. 4:23) and this must be checked before injection of large quantities of local anaesthetic. Simple aspiration may reveal the intravenous placement (Fig. 4:24) but this is not totally reliable as the negative pressure applied may suck the vein wall against the end of the catheter and obstruct it. It is best to lower the protruding end below the patient's spine and allow any blood to escape by gravity. If frank blood is seen, the catheter must be removed and reinserted. If bloodstained fluid is seen, the catheter or needle may or may not be in a vein. A test dose as described below may then be useful in determing the location of the catheter or needle.

Fig. 4:23 Catheter lying within an epidural vein.

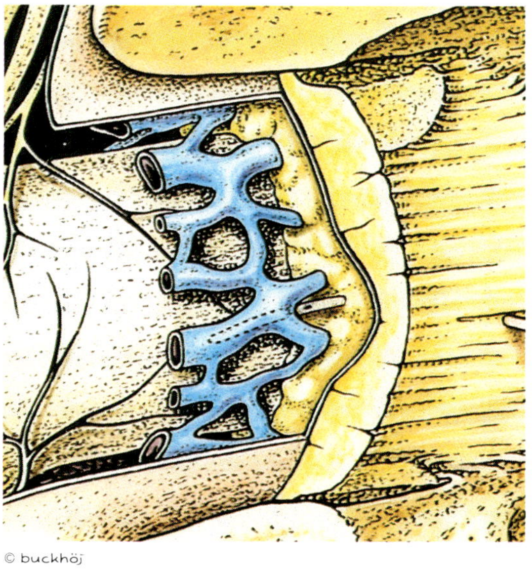

Fig. 4:24 Aspiration of blood along catheter.

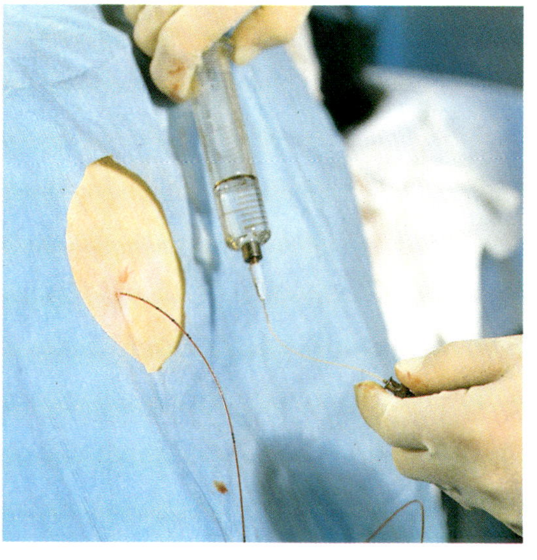

Drugs and dosage

Test dose

Before injecting the chosen dose of drug, many anaesthetists prefer to inject a small test dose to eliminate the possibility of the needle or catheter being in a vein or within the subarachnoid space.

The amount of drug used as a test dose and the time allowed must be adequate to show the effects of incorrect placement. Thus 4-5 ml of drug injected into the subarachnoid space and left for 5 min will give an easily detected spinal block, whereas 2 ml left for 2 min might well not do so. Two ml of a hyperbaric spinal solution will show most quickly that a subarachnoid injection has been made, but will have very little effect in the epidural space, unlike say 5 ml of 2% lidocaine or 0.5% bupivacaine, which may produce a block over several spinal segments. If the needle or catheter is lying within a vein, even 5 ml may be insufficient to cause systemic effects unless epinephrine (0.1 mg, i.e. 0.1 ml of 1:1000 solution) is added and the heart rate and arterial pressure are measured before and after injection. *It is important that if a test dose is used, a negative result should not be taken as absolute proof of correct placement, and care must still be taken while injecting the main dose.* If a test dose has been given through the needle, a further test dose should be given after insertion of the catheter.

Main dose

Many drugs can be used for epidural block and a full account of these is given in Chap. 3. Because of the size and thickness of the coverings of the spinal nerves, drugs must be used in high concentration for complete nerve blockade, though weaker solutions may be used for pain relief; this is especially so when the pain is mediated through autonomic nerves, as is the pain of labour.

The volume to be used will depend upon the required height of blockade (see Chap. 5) and the general condition of the patient. The spread of fluid within the epidural space is not linearly related to the volume injected. Ten ml of solution injected at L_2-L_3 will reach most of the space up to T_9-T_7. A further 10 ml will only raise this to T_7-T_5 on average. As a result of this, when 20 ml has been used, each spinal nerve is affected by a greater amount of drug, leading to a more profound and prolonged blockade.

The simplest approach to dosage is to plan on injecting rather more than is thought necessary to block nerves to the required level. Thus failure to achieve an adequate height will be greatly reduced and more prolonged blockade will result. Unduly high blocks are uncommon and if properly managed will cause little upset to patients unless they are either very old or very ill. With a catheter, dosage can be varied at will according to the response to the initial injection.

Because the total dose of the drug is likely to cause toxic effects if given rapidly into an epidural vein, it is important to inject slowly (10 $ml.min^{-1}$) even though the test dose gave a negative result. An alternative approach is to inject the local anaesthetic in small aliquots, e.g., 5 ml every 5 min until the necessary height of blockade is achieved.

For surgical procedures, the following dosage will be adequate in most patients, but it may have to be modified depending on the clinical situation:

Abdominal surgery: 15-25 ml of the following: 2% lidocaine, 2% prilocaine or 2% mepivacaine, 0.5%-0.75% bupivacaine, 1.0% -1.5% etidocaine. While the lower concentrations often give satisfactory results, the higher are more reliable and give a longer duration.

Lower limb, hip and perineal surgery: 10-15 ml of similar concentrations.

Epinephrine: epinephrine 1:200,000 will increase the intensity and duration of the block, though this will depend upon the drug used (see page 73).

Analgesia: for analgesia, bupivacaine is the agent of choice because of its long duration and sparing effect on motor nerves. The dosage for the relief of labour pain is usually 6-10 ml of 0.25%-0.5%. Uterine contractions are relieved by blockade of T_{10}-L_1 segments. Perineal pain in the second and third stages requires blockade of S_2-S_4 (see page 119).

For postoperative pain relief the best results are obtained when the catheter tip is placed at or near the centre of the band of anaesthesia required. Only a few segments need to be blocked, e.g., T_8-T_{12} for a lower abdominal operation or L_1-L_3 for a hip operation. Small quantities of local anaesthetic may be used but must be given frequently, e.g., 4-5 ml of 0.5% bupivacaine hourly. Alternatively a continuous infusion of 15-25 $ml.hour^{-1}$ of 0.1% or 0.125% bupivacaine, gives good results (see p. 126).

Thoracic epidural block

Lumbar epidural block is the most commonly used epidural technique because it is relatively easy and the needle is inserted below the termination of the spinal cord. Its disadvantage is that considerable volumes of solution have to be injected to reach the mid-thoracic nerves. Moreover there is inevitably blockade of the lumbar and sacral nerves. During abdominal operations, this is of little importance, but if the blockade is to be prolonged into the postoperative period for pain relief then the paralysis of the legs and perineum, together with the loss of sacral autonomic function (micturition, control of sphincters, etc.), presents problems for both patients and nursing staff.

If the epidural catheter can be placed at a point in the middle of the required band of analgesia, then much less drug can be used and unnecessary blockade of other nerves is prevented. The abdomen is supplied by the thoracic segments T_6 to T_{12}. To be at the centre of the required band of analgesia, the spinal canal must be entered through the thoracic intervertebral spaces, T_{10}-T_{11} or T_{11}-T_{12} for lower abdominal operations and T_7-T_8 or T_8-T_9 for upper abdominal operations. Even higher blocks can be used for thoracic operations to provide postoperative pain relief. Thoracic epidurals are also commonly used for relieving the pain due to multiple fractured ribs.

Anatomical and technical considerations

The spinous processes of the thoracic vertebrae vary considerably in their angulation. The 1st, 2nd, 10th, 11th and 12th are, like the lumbar vertebrae, almost horizontal in the sagittal plane and allow a needle to be inserted at or near 90° to the skin. The other thoracic spinous processes are angled downwards to a greater or lesser extent and this requires a different technique to ensure entrance into the epidural space.

Entering the epidural space between T_{10}-T_{11}, T_{11}-T_{12} or T_{12}-L_1 is easy and can be performed exactly as for lumbar epidural block. Because the spinous processes of T_{10}, T_{11} and T_{12} are shorter than those of the lumbar vertebrae, the spinal canal is at a lesser depth from the skin. The needle should be inserted at right angles and loss of resistance, as the ligamentum flavum is penetrated, will be easily determined.

It might be thought that it would be relatively easy to direct the catheter upwards and advance it to a higher level in the epidural space. However, this is very unpredictable and the tip of the catheter may double back on itself. Thus if a high placement is required there is no substitute for inserting the needle at the appropriate interspace.

Two techniques are possible for midthoracic blocks, a midline or a paramedian approach.

Midline approach

A needle inserted between the spinous processes in the midline has to be directed at an angle of about 45° to the skin so as to pass parallel to the spinous processes above and below (Fig. 4:25). The area of the ligamentum flavum accessible at this angle is rather less than with the right-angled approach lower down the spine. If bone is contacted and prevents the onward movement, then the anaesthetist must manipulate the needle so that it misses bone and continues on into the spinal canal. In most instances this can be accomplished without difficulty. Experience with a considerable number of lumbar epidural blocks is an advantage provided the more superficial position of the spinal canal is appreciated.

Paramedian or lateral approach

In the mid-thoracic region not only are the spinous processes very angulated, but also the laminae tend to overlap each other. Thus the paramedian approach though avoiding the spinous processes has to be at a relatively acute angle to negotiate the space between the laminae, which, of course, is occupied by the ligamentum flavum. The needle is inserted 1-1.5 cm from the upper border of the spinous process below the chosen interspace at an even more acute angle than in the midline approach. It is aimed medially but should avoid contact with the spinous processes. If bone is contacted, it will therefore be the lamina, and the needle must be redirected to negotiate the space between the laminae.

The anaesthetist should have a good three-dimensional sense of the vertebral anatomy, and inspection of a skeleton helps considerably.

Fig. 4:25 Thoracic epidural injection, showing angulation of the needle so as to be parallel to the spinous processes.

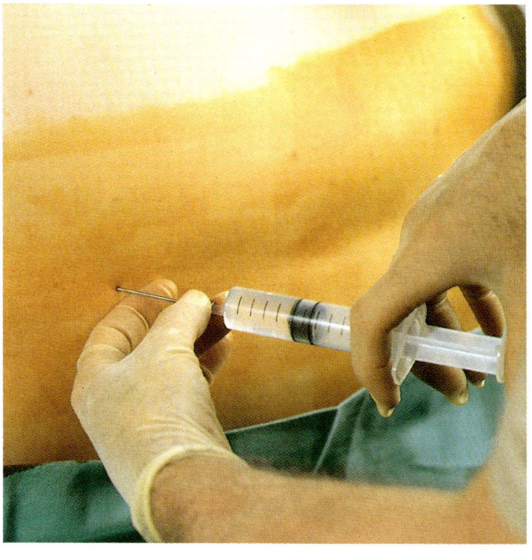

Fig. 4:26 Entry of the needle into the thoracic epidural space. Note the position of the point in relation to the dura mater.

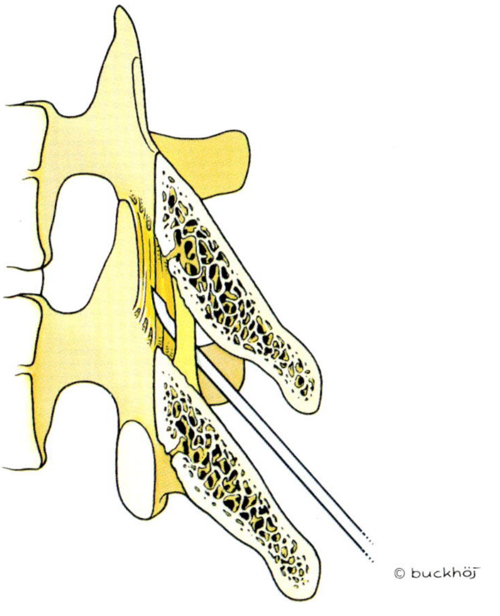

Because of the angulation of the needle, either with the midline or the lateral approach, the epidural space is entered at an acute angle with the curved end of the Tuohy needle nearest the dura (Fig. 4:26). Puncture of the dura is therefore less likely than with the horizontal approach in the lower thoracic or lumbar areas. Moreover the insertion of the catheter is easy and it will move cephalad without obstruction. The Crawford needle (see p. 87) may have particular advantages in this regard.

Dosage

Abdominal surgery

For abdominal surgery 10-15 ml of the higher concentration of local anaesthetics will give good results.

For pain relief

3 - 5 ml of concentrated local anaesthetic solution will block 2 to 4 segments above and below the tip of the catheter. Thus dosage should be on a trial and error basis initially, but repeated doses are very consistent in their behaviour.

Small volume (and therefore small dose) injections have a shorter duration of action than larger ones and it is therefore necessary to repeat them every 1-2 h as necessary. Where prolonged pain relief is required, an automatic pump delivering small bolus injections is valuable. Otherwise a constant infusion of dilute solution (e.g., 0.125% bupivacaine at 10 - 20 $ml.hour^{-1}$) gives satisfactory results.

Cervical epidural block

This is very occasionally used to provide analgesia in chronic pain states, though it has been used for thoracic, thyroid and breast surgery. Access to the cervical epidural space is relatively easy, but great care must be taken to avoid direct trauma to the spinal cord. The C_7-T_1 interspace is the widest and easiest space to use.

The cervical spinous processes are not angulated and a horizontal approach is indicated (Fig. 4:27). The ligamentum flavum is thin and will be reached quite superficially. The needle should be advanced with the greatest care. The usual loss of resistance will be easily appreciated. It is advised that only anaesthetists with considerable experience of lumbar epidural block should undertake this procedure.

Dosage

On average 10 ml of local anaesthetic will block the spinal nerves from C_4 to T_8. The more concentrated local anaesthetics may cause motor blockade of C_2, C_3 and C_4, with paralysis of the diaphragm. Thus the less potent concentrations (1%-1.5% lidocaine, 0.5% bupivacaine) are indicated.

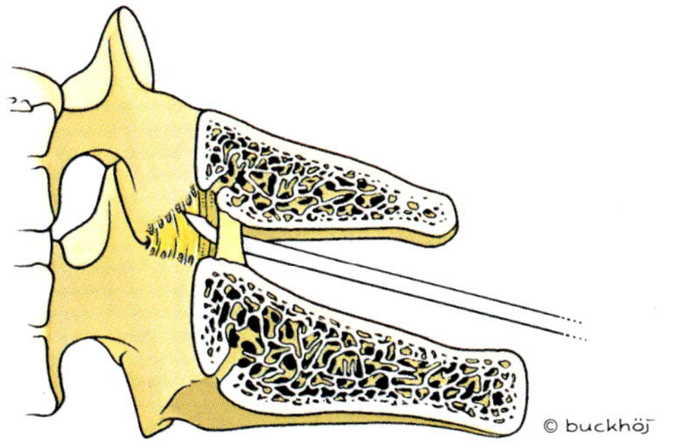

Fig. 4:27 Cervical epidural puncture. Note that the spinous processes are almost horizontal.

Caudal block

Because the epidural space ends at the lower end of the sacrum it is possible to enter it through the sacral hiatus, thus greatly reducing the possibility of a dural tap because the subarachnoid space ends at the level of S_2. The patient may be placed laterally, or prone with a pillow under the pelvis.

The sacral hiatus is palpated using the sacral cornuae as the landmarks (Fig. 4:28). The skin is cleaned and the patient draped as for lumbar epidural block. An intradermal wheal is raised with local anaesthetic over the sacral hiatus (Fig. 4:29). A needle is then inserted at 45° to the sacro-coccygeal ligament which is pierced and the anterior wall of the sacral canal contacted (Fig. 4:30). The needle may then be redirected so that it is more in line with the spinal canal (Fig 4:31a and b), and advanced 1 - 2 mm into the canal (Fig 4:32).

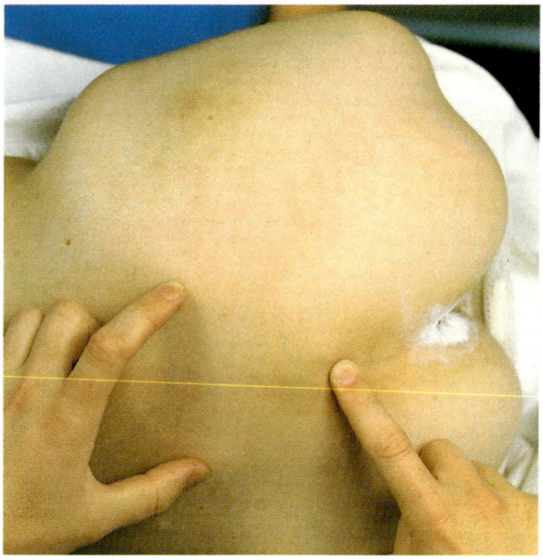

Fig. 4:28

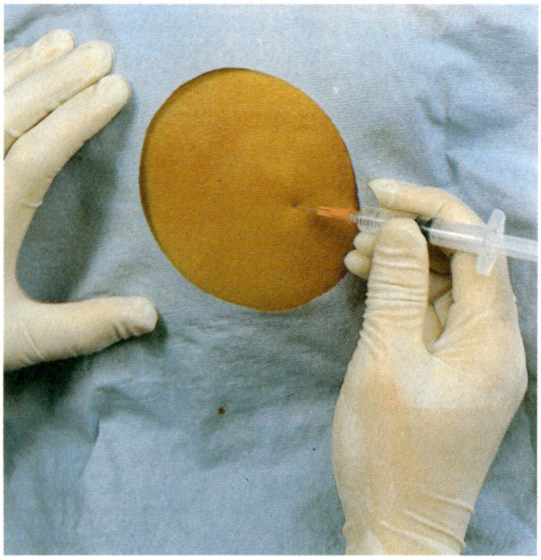

Fig. 4:29

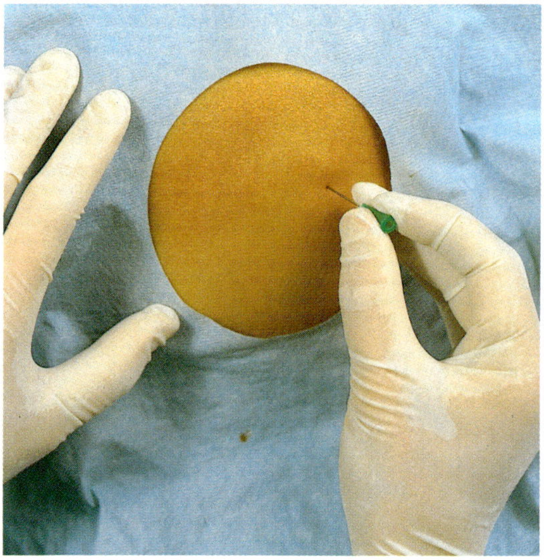

Fig. 4:30

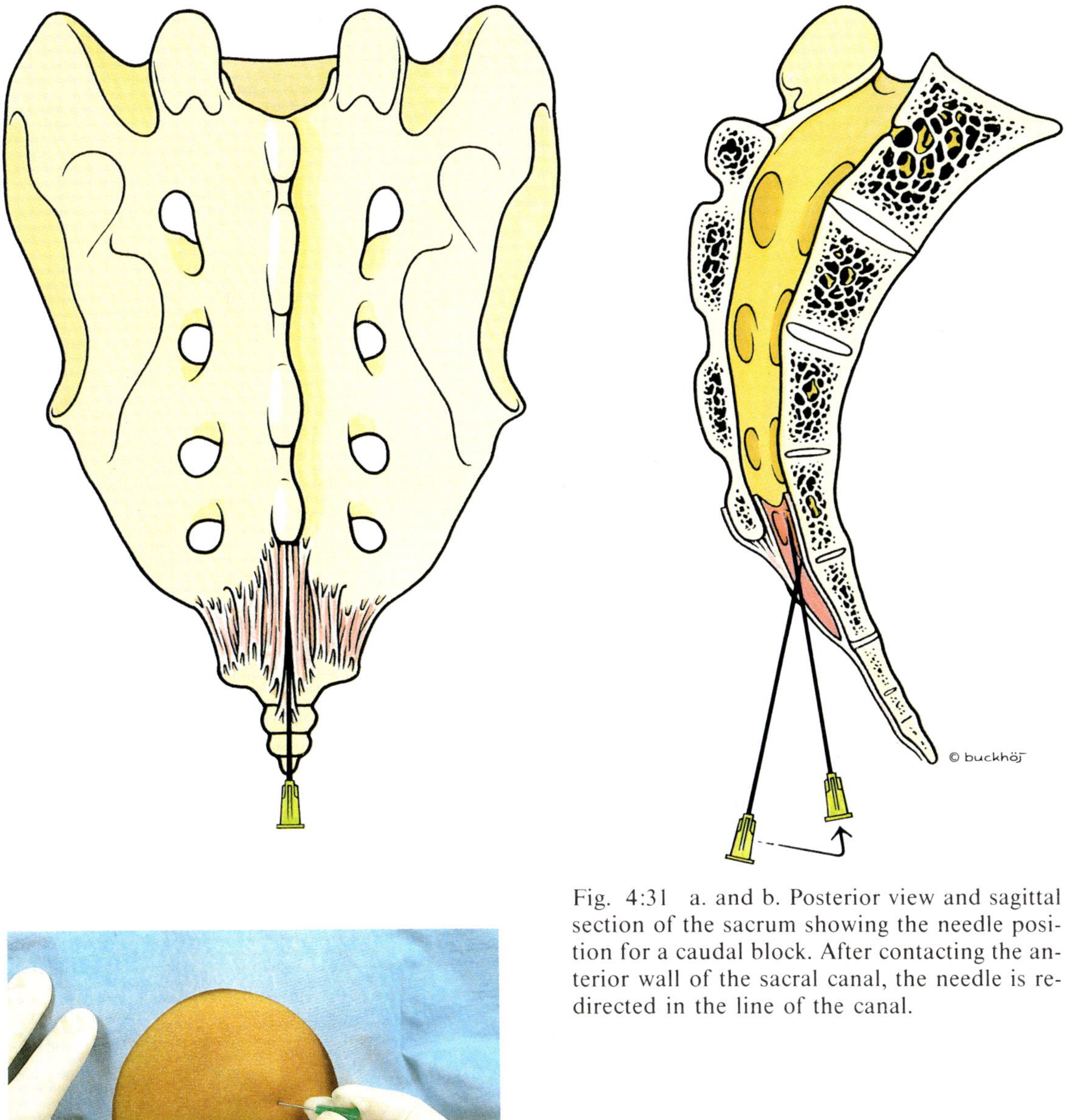

Fig. 4:31 a. and b. Posterior view and sagittal section of the sacrum showing the needle position for a caudal block. After contacting the anterior wall of the sacral canal, the needle is redirected in the line of the canal.

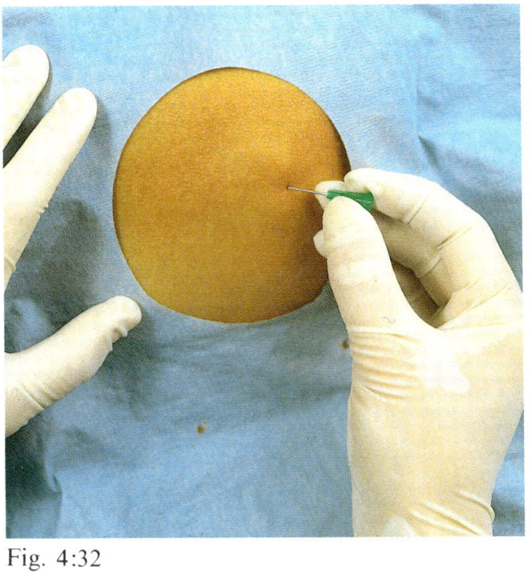

Fig. 4:32

Various needles are available for caudal block, but a simple 4 cm, 21-23 gauge disposable needle is all that is required. If a catheter is being used, the needle must of course be of sufficiently large bore (16-18 gauge) to allow the catheter to pass through its lumen.

Injection of local anaesthetic is then made, observing the skin over the sacrum (Fig. 4:33). Should subcutaneous swelling occur, this would indicate a wrongly placed injection.

A finger palpating the sacrococcygeal ligament during the initial injection will feel the ligament bulging outwards, thus confirming accurate placement.

Dosage

Because the injection is made at one end of the epidural space rather than near the middle, it is more difficult to achieve spread into the thoracic region. Thus higher volumes of local anaesthetic are required than with lumbar epidural block.

For adults it requires 20 ml to ensure blockade of the sacral nerves. Thirty millilitres is usually required to ensure spread into the lower thoracic area. The most concentrated solutions are required for surgery.

A test dose (see p. 98) can be used to diagnose intravascular placement of the needle.

Indications

Theoretically caudal block can be used for any indication recommended for lumbar epidural block. However, there is often difficulty in getting the local anaesthetic to spread high enough. As a result the technique is generally reserved for procedures which require blockade of the sacral nerves, though the lumbar and lower thoracic nerves can usually be blocked with the appropriate dosage. Thus the main indications are:

1. Perineal operations
2. Inguinal and femoral herniorrhaphy
3. Cystoscopy and urethral surgery

Caudal block was widely used for relief of pain in labour but has been largely replaced by lumbar epidurals.

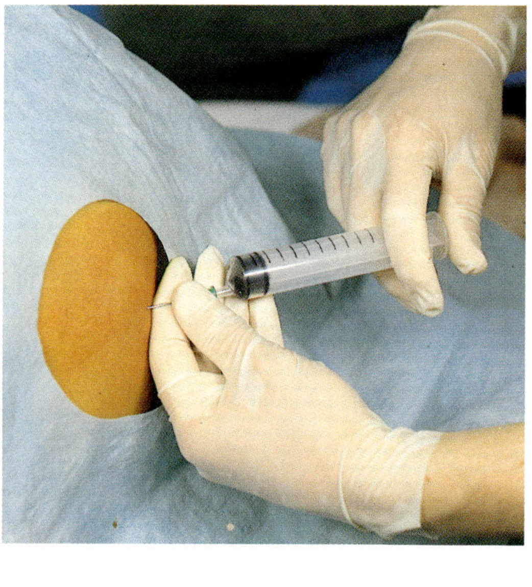

Fig. 4:33 The skin over the sacral hiatus is observed during injection.

Caudal block in paediatric surgery

Caudal block is quite easy to perform in children and has achieved popularity in operations such as herniorrhaphy, circumcision etc. It is usual to give the patient a light general anaesthetic before carrying out the block.

Dosage in children

In the literature there are widely differing recommendations given for the dosage of local anaesthetic to be used for caudal block in children. Most of the operations performed require nerve blocks to the height of T_{10} or below.

It takes relatively small doses of local anaesthetic to achieve this level of block. Greater amounts will cause much higher blocks, but the disadvantage of this will not be apparent because children respond much less to widespread sympathetic blockade than do adults. In addition high systemic concentrations of local anaesthetics will not produce overt toxicity due to the concomitant use of general anaesthesia in these children. Thus considerable variations in dosage will have little effect upon the end result. Nevertheless, the use of excessive doses should be avoided. The recommendations given below have been set towards the lower end of the doses to be found in the literature.

There are two ways of calculating the dose, one based on body weight and the other on age. In normal sized children, either method can be used successfully, even though the relationship between age and weight is not linear. However if the child is obese then there is a danger of overdosage and it is better to use age rather than body weight. Conversely if the patient is obviously bigger or smaller than the average for age, then the body weight should be used.

The two drugs most commonly used are lidocaine 1% and bupivacaine 0.25%. The choice lies in the desired duration of effect. The doses given below are therefore in millilitres and are the same for both drugs.

Age	Dose (ml) for block to	
(yrs)	T_{12}	T_7
2	4	6
3	5	7.5
4	5.5	8
5	6	9
6	7	10.5
7	8	12
8	9	13.5
9	10	15
10	11	16.5

Body weight	Dose (ml) for block to	
(Kg)	T_{12}	T_7
10	3	4.5
12.5	4	6
15	5	7.5
17.5	6	9
20	7	10.5
22.5	8	12
25	9	13.5
27.5	10	15
30	11	16.5

References & Bibliography

Armitage, E.N. (1979). Caudal block in children. Anaesthesia 34, 396.

Bromage. P.R. (1978). Epidural Analgesia. Saunders Co., Philadelphia.

Cousins. M.J. (1980). Epidural neural blockade. Neural Blockade Eds.

Cousins. M.J. & Bridenbaugh, P.O. J.B. Lippincott Co., Philadelphia p. 176.

Lee. J.A. & Atkinson. R.S. (1978). Sir Robert Macintosh' Lumbar Puncture and Spinal Analgesia. Churchill Livingstone. Edinburgh.

McCaul. K. (1980). Caudal blockade. Neural blockade, Eds. Cousins, M.J. & Bridenbaugh, P.O. J.B. Lippincott & Co., Philadelphia p. 275.

Schulte-Steinberg. O. & Ralps, V.W. (1977). Spread of extradural analgesia following caudal injection in children: a statistical study. Brit. J. Anaesth 49. 1027.

5. Clinical considerations

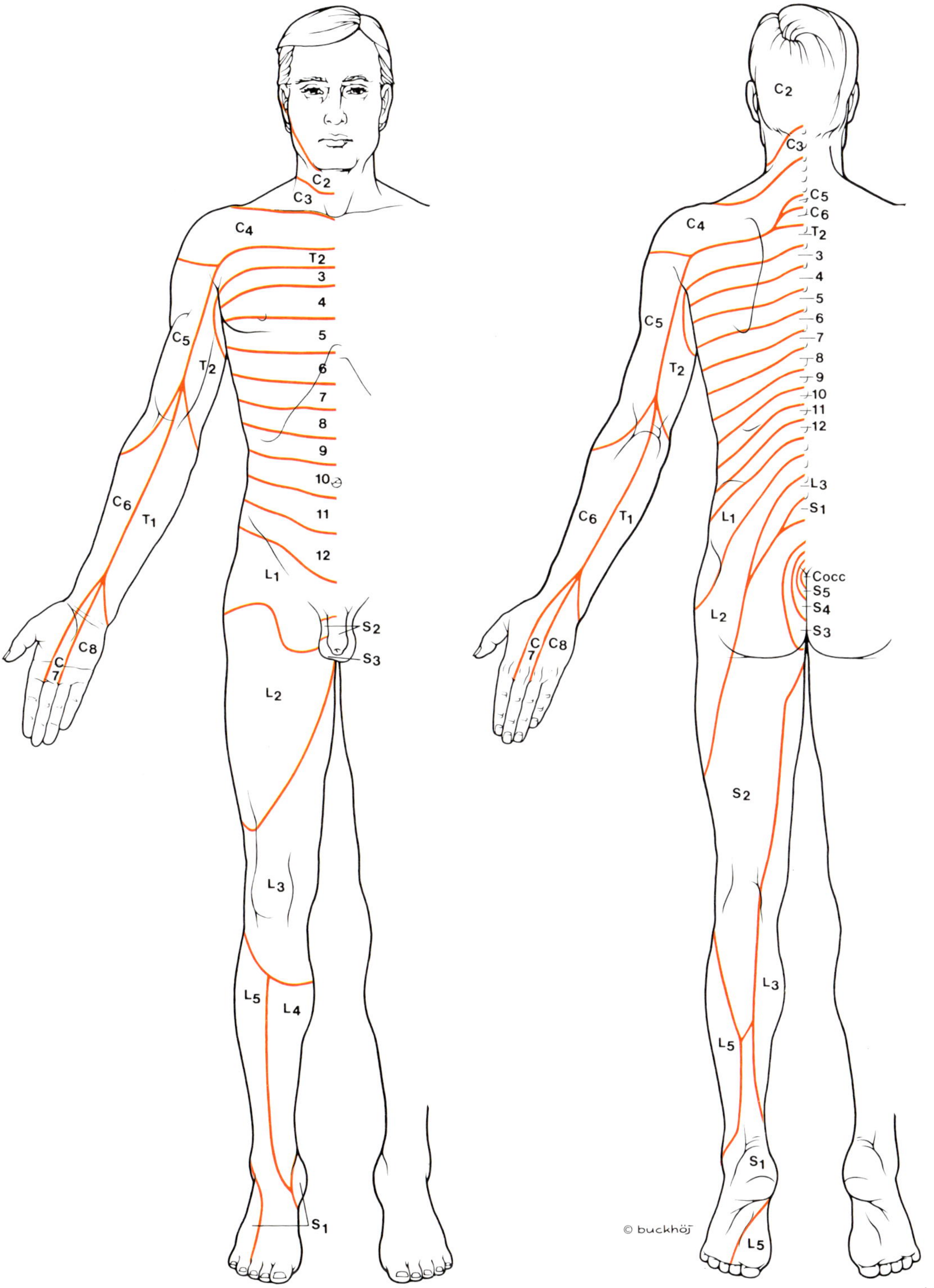

The clinical use of epidural block will be discussed under the following headings:

1. **Surgery**
2. **Obstetrics**
3. **Acute pain**
4. **Chronic pain**

Epidural block in surgery

Advantages

Epidural blockade has many advantages over general anaesthesia when performed for surgical operations.

Because all modalities of nerve function (sensory, motor and autonomic) are affected by epidural block, it can be used to provide complete anaesthesia during surgical operations. All sensory input from the operation can be obtunded and muscle relaxation provided at the operative site

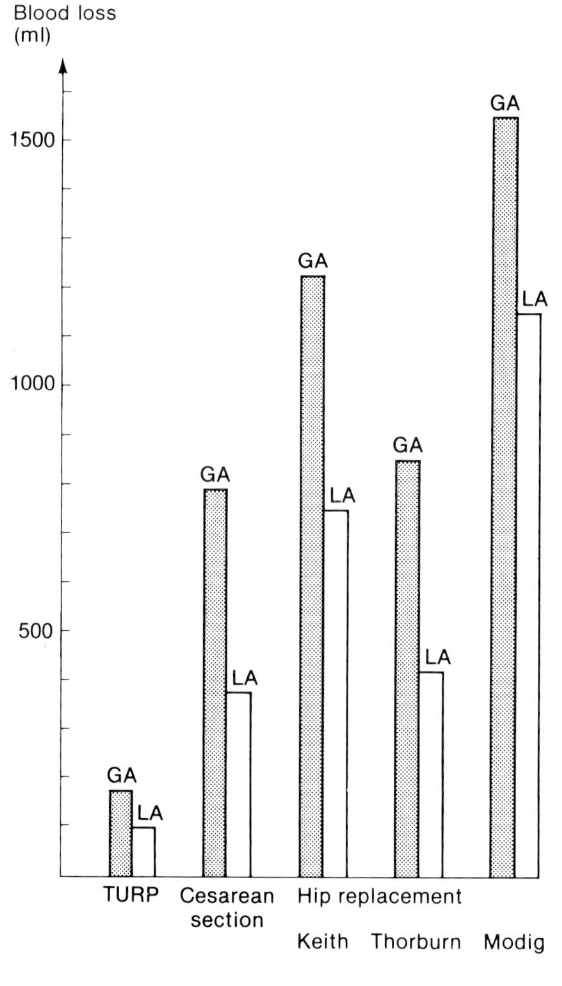

Fig. 5:1 Reduction in blood loss in patients receiving epidural block.

and not in *all* voluntary muscles, as is the case with relaxants. Because of this, spontaneous respiration is unaffected, as are the upper airway reflexes. Even with concomitant general anaesthesia, spontaneous respiration can be maintained and there is seldom any need to intubate the trachea. Thus the problems of sympathetic stimulation producing hypertension and tachycardia during intubation and surgery almost never occur. Spontaneous breathing offers one of the best monitors during anaesthesia. It allows judgement of the adequacy of the airway, gaseous exchange, depth of anaesthesia and cerebral circulation.

There is considerable evidence that operative blood loss is reduced in patients receiving epidural block, particularly in operations such as prostatectomy, Caesarean section, hip replacement (Fig. 5:1) and radical pelvic surgery. This is related in part to the reduction in arterial pressure that often occurs and to reduced venous pressure.

Fig. 5:2 Reduction in the incidence of deep venous thrombosis and pulmonary embolus in patients receiving epidural block.

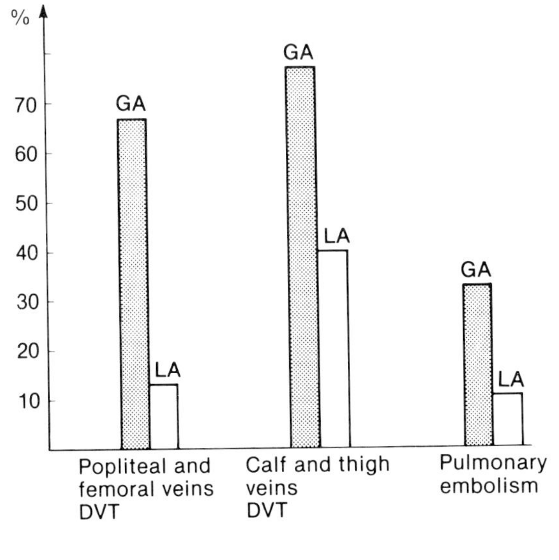

Large bowel anastomoses have been shown to heal better with fewer breakdowns. Sacral parasympathetic block reduces bowel motility while sympathetic block increases blood flow to the bowel and these contribute to optimal healing.

Postoperatively there is a reduction in the incidence of deep venous thrombosis and pulmonary embolus (Fig. 5:2). This is probably related to the increased blood flow in the legs due to the sympathetic blockade.

Fig. 5:3 Blood flow through femoral artery grafts in patients anaesthetised either with epidural anaesthesia followed by continuous epidural block postoperatively, or with general anaesthesia and opioids postoperatively.

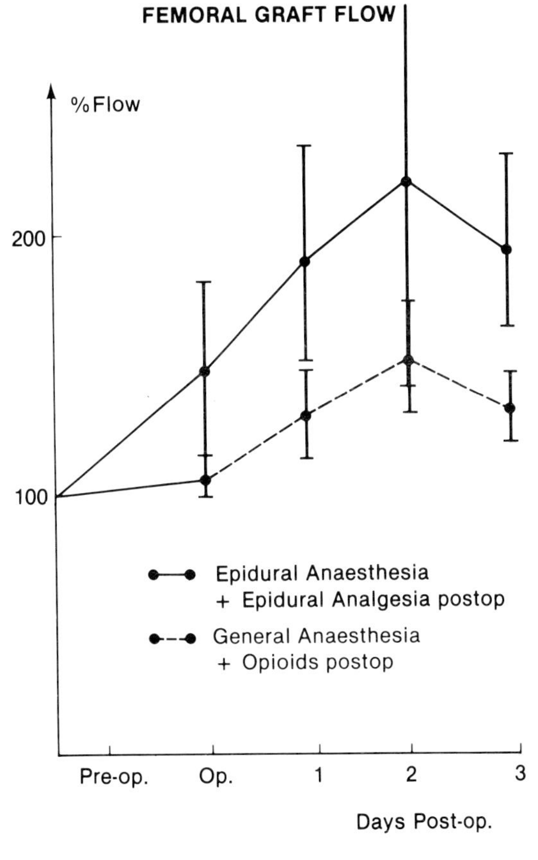

Fig. 5:4 Changes during the perioperative period in
a. Fibrinolysis inhibition (using dilution of amino-caproic acid)
b. Plasmaingen activators
c. Factor VIII capacity
From Brit. J. Anaesth. (1983) Vol. 55 p 625.
Reprinted by permission of the author.

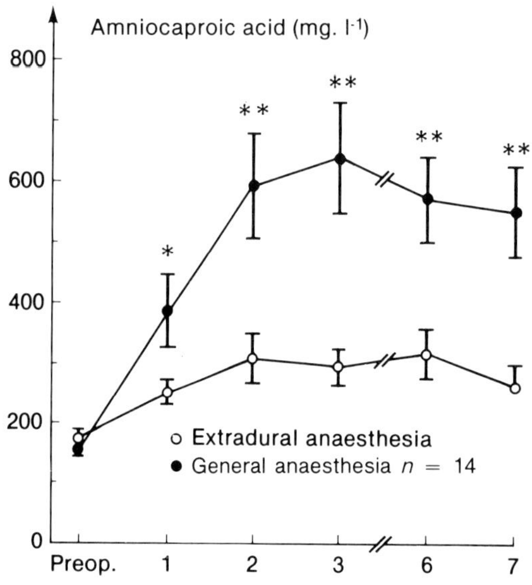

Fig. 5:4a

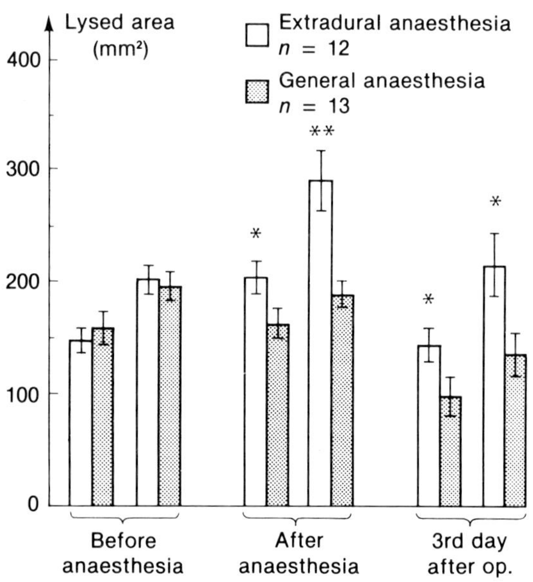

Fig. 5:4b

In cases of femoral artery bypass, blood flow through the graft is significantly greater when epidural block is used and continued into the postoperative period, compared with general anaesthesia and analgesia with opioid drugs. (Fig. 5:3).

In addition, the local anaesthetic drugs themselves may influence thrombus formation and fibrinolytic activity (Fig. 5:4a-c).

Even minor trauma to the endothelium of veins results in vigorous activity by leucocytes which penetrate the lining cells and can initiate thrombus formation. This activity can be considerably reduced by intravenous infusions of lidocaine (Fig. 5:5a and b).

The ability to control postoperative pain allows the patient to move and breathe without discomfort and prevents the sympathetic overactivity sometimes seen with severe pain. The avoidance of large doses of opioids encourages early recovery of gastrointestinal function. It also prevents respiratory depression and airway obstruction during sleep.

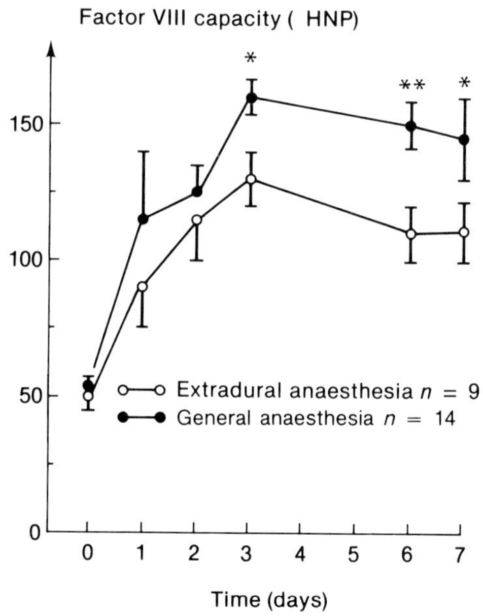

Fig. 5:4c

Fig. 5:5 a. Electron micrograph of a canine jugular vein subjected to a brief period of occlusion. Note adherence and invasion of endothelium by leucocytes. b. Similar vein in a dog receiving i.v. lidocaine showing considerable modifications in the leucocyte reaction.
From Regional Anesthesia, (1982) Supplement Vol. 7, No 4.
Reprinted by permission of the author.

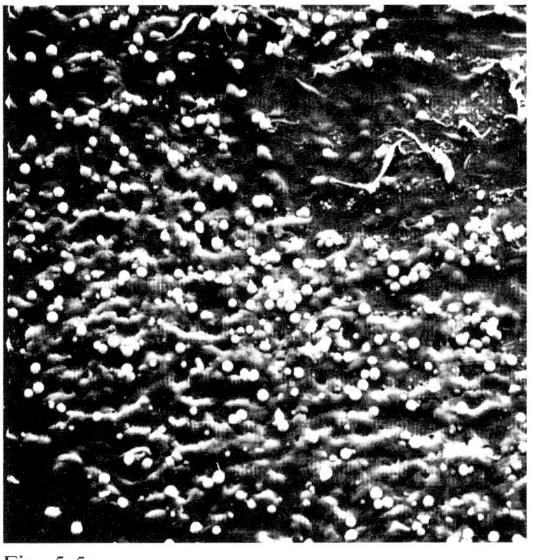

Fig. 5:5a

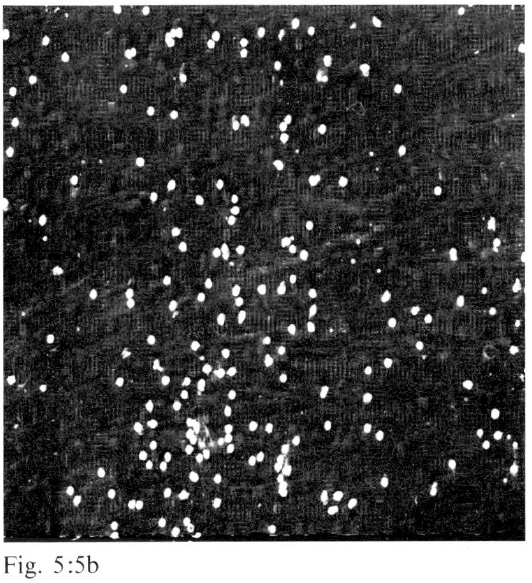

Fig. 5:5b

The reduction in surgical stress that derives from afferent blockade helps in the patient's well-being and speed of recovery.

To summarise, the advantages of epidural block in surgery are:

a. Reduction in surgical stress
b. Retention of spontaneous breathing and upper airway reflexes
c. Reduced blood loss
d. Better healing of bowel anastomoses
e. Better postoperative pain control
f. Reduced incidence of thromboembolism
g. Quicker recovery of gastrointestinal function

Indications

Abdominal surgery

Lower abdominal operations are particularly suitable for epidural anaesthesia, especially those involving large bowel, bladder, prostate, and the female reproductive organs.

Upper abdominal surgery, though less popular, can be performed under epidural block but steps must be taken to reduce the effects of vagal stimulation as the vagus nerves are unaffected by the blockade. The easiest way to do this is to use a concomitant general anaesthetic of appropriate depth.

Vaginal and perineal surgery

For these operations epidural block offers excellent operating conditions with reduced blood loss. The intense afferent stimulation associated with operations on the perineum is totally removed by the sacral nerve blockade. Relaxation of the anal sphincter also helps with operations at that site.

Urological surgery

Virtually all urological operations can be performed under epidural blockade. This includes operations on the kidney, though the anaesthetist must be wary of accidental opening of the pleural cavity in a spontaneously breathing patient.

Lower limb surgery

All such operations will benefit from the use of epidural anaesthesia, with particularly good results in hip replacement and vascular surgery.

Management of surgical patients during epidural anaesthesia

Many operations performed under epidural block are major ones and some form of sedation is usually required. This can vary in degree from light sedation to general anaesthesia and will be dictated by circumstances. Many patients prefer to be asleep and the use of general anaesthesia does not preclude the use of epidural block. Indeed, there is good evidence that the combination of light general anaesthesia with epidural block offers the most complete protection from surgical stress during surgery.

In other circumstances the patient may wish to be awake. In Caesarean sections not only can the mother be awake during the birth of her baby, but also sedative drugs depressant to the foetus can be avoided until the umbilical cord is clamped.

The attitude of the whole surgical team is important to success if patients are to remain awake. Nurses, surgeons and anaesthetists must be sympathetic and supportive, and refrain from making remarks which can alarm the patient. The surgeon must work with reasonable gentleness and speed. Should the patient experience discomfort, the anaesthetist must be able to give reassurance and offer positive help in the form of analgesics.

Premedication

This is usually given an hour before surgery and the oral or intramuscular routes are the most commonly used. Personal preference will dictate whether an opioid or a sedative or both is used. If general anaesthesia is to be used, an antisialogogue such as atropine is useful.

Sedative drugs

A wide range of drugs can be used to sedate patients and they may be divided into sedatives and analgesics. Sedatives are indicated if the patient is nervous. If, on the other hand, the epidural block is less than totally effective, an analgesic drug will be more suitable. Opioids are ideal for this purpose as they have sedative properties as well as being effective analgesics. A patient experiencing some pain or discomfort should not be given a sedative alone since these drugs frequently cause the patient to become quite uncooperative if the pain is not relieved.

Generally speaking it should be possible to give sedative drugs intravenously and the shorter the duration of action of the drugs the better. Most anaesthetists will have their favourite drugs, and no list is likely to be complete. Among the sedatives are:

- Benzodiazepines, e.g., diazepam, temazepam and midazolam. These are generally given by intermittent intravenous doses. They have relatively long half-lives and are potent amnesics. They are also respiratory depressants.

- Short-acting hypnotic drugs given by continuous intravenous infusion, such as thiopental, methohexitone, and chlormethiazole. The patient can be kept well sedated but is often rousable. If they are given for a long time, accumulation can occur and lead to long-lasting sedation. Generally their effect can be well controlled by the rate of infusion and recovery is rapid at the end of surgery.

Analgesic drugs

Opioids in particular are widely used during epidural block and are indicated if analgesia is less than perfect. Medium-acting drugs include morphine, diamorphine and pethidine. Short-acting drugs such as fentanyl are also available. Usually they are given by intermittent intravenous injection, although it may be more logical to give a continuous infusion so as to maintain a steady state.

General anaesthesia

This, provided it is light and simple, offers many advantages, such as:

- The patient often prefers to be asleep, particularly if the operation is lengthy.

- It speeds up the whole process considerably in that the patient can be prepared for surgery before the block is fully developed.

- The analgesia associated with light general anaesthesia ensures that any minor deficiency in the epidural block is not felt by the patient.

- It provides the maximum reduction of surgical stress.

- It allows the use of induced hypotension, which is unpleasant in the conscious patient who may react by vasovagal fainting when the arterial pressure decreases. General anaesthesia facilitates the reduction in arterial pressure.

- Anaesthesia is easily and quickly controlled in regard to depth and duration, all the inhalational agents having very short half-lives.

The drugs used will again largely depend upon the preference of the anaesthetist. An intravenous agent such as thiopental, or methohexital may be used for induction.

Anaesthesia can be maintained with inhalational agents (nitrous oxide, halothane, enflurane, isoflurane, etc). Deep anaesthesia is not required and spontaneous respiration is maintained with advantage. As with all forms of general anaesthesia, care of the airway is of prime importance. Endotracheal intubation is seldom required except in upper abdominal surgery or in operations when patient position can make airway control difficult.

Peri-operative management

Monitoring of the heart rate, arterial pressure and ECG are essential. Unconscious patients must also be observed in regard to their airway and breathing. Quiet regular breathing will indicate that the patient has a satisfactory block and is asleep. Apnoea may be due to too light a plane of anaesthesia, obstructed airway, respiratory depression or circulatory arrest.

Hypotension

Hypotension should be treated promptly unless it is to be induced for surgical reasons. Preloading the patient with 500 - 1000 ml of crystalloid solution is usually effective in preventing hypotension. If it should occur, it is better to use a vasopressor drug (e.g., ephedrine 15 mg) which will produce a rapid effect (sometimes it requires more than one injection) regardless of whether the hypotension is due to sympathetic blockade, vasovagal fainting or both. Alternatively a drug such as phenylephrine can be given by i.v. infusion, the dose being titrated to the patient's blood pressure response. Hypotension is discussed in greater detail on p. 158.

Induced hypotension

Induced hypotension to reduce operative bleeding should only be used in patients receiving general anaesthesia combined with the epidural block. It is especially indicated in radical surgery involving considerable blood loss (radical hysterectomy, abdomino-perineal resection of the rectum, etc.) but is also useful in less major operations (e.g., vaginal repairs) where even small amounts of blood can obscure the operative field.

Postoperative care

Patients who have had epidural blocks will usually regain their mental faculties quickly if deep sedation has been avoided. Even when general anaesthesia has been added, the patient awakens quickly and recovers all reflexes necessary for maintenance of the airway, usually before the onset of postoperative pain.

The blood pressure tends to be somewhat labile for an hour or so after surgery, though hypotension seldom causes any problem. If it is considered that the pressure is too low, it may be increased quickly and easily. Raising the foot of the bed prevents pooling of blood in dependent veins. The intravenous infusion of crystalloid 250 - 500 ml given over 15 - 30 min will often increase the arterial pressure to acceptable levels. In severe cases or when a rapid response is required, a vasopressor, e.g., ephedrine (15 mg), may be given intravenously and repeated if necessary. An intramuscular injection of the same dose of vasopressor at the same time as the intravenous dose will maintain the pressure over a longer period. It is very unusual to have to resort to vasopressors in a patient more than once. Indeed, in such cases an alternative cause for the hypotension, such as haemorrhage, should be sought.

The epidural block may be continued into the postoperative period for pain relief (vide infra). If it is not, the block will sooner or later wear off and the patient will require normal postoperative care. As the legs may remain numb and paralysed for some time, the patient should be reassured that recovery will be complete. Attention to pressure points with changes in posture may be required if the block is prolonged.

Contra-indications

These are few but include:

- Patients with blood coagulation problems. There is a risk of causing an epidural haematoma if the patient's blood is hypocoagulable during insertion of the epidural needle or catheter. Whether this is the case with patients who are given anticoagulants after insertion of the catheter is still contested and the exact degree of risk is not known. However, several studies involving thousands of patients have been reported and have not shown any undue risk in these circumstances. This also applies to patients receiving "mini-dose" heparin to prevent deep venous thrombosis. The risk of thrombosis is in any case considerably reduced by epidural block and the need for heparin prophylaxis is likewise reduced.

- Active infection in the area of needle and catheter insertion.

- Severe hypovolaemia. In such patients the elimination of sympathetic circulatory control can lead to profound hypotension and circulatory collapse.

- Active neurological disease is considered by many to be a contra-indication, though there is no evidence that epidural block can adversely affect the course of such disease.

Epidural block in obstetric analgesia and anaesthesia

It is in the field of obstetrics that epidural block has become most popular. It is by far the most effective means of relieving pain in labour and it allows the performance of a Caesarean section on a conscious mother.

Originally, epidural block in labour was performed mainly by the caudal route, but this has largely given way to the lumbar approach.

The insertion of the epidural needle and catheter is not different in the pregnant patient but there are important differences in regard to the block required and to the physiological changes it causes.

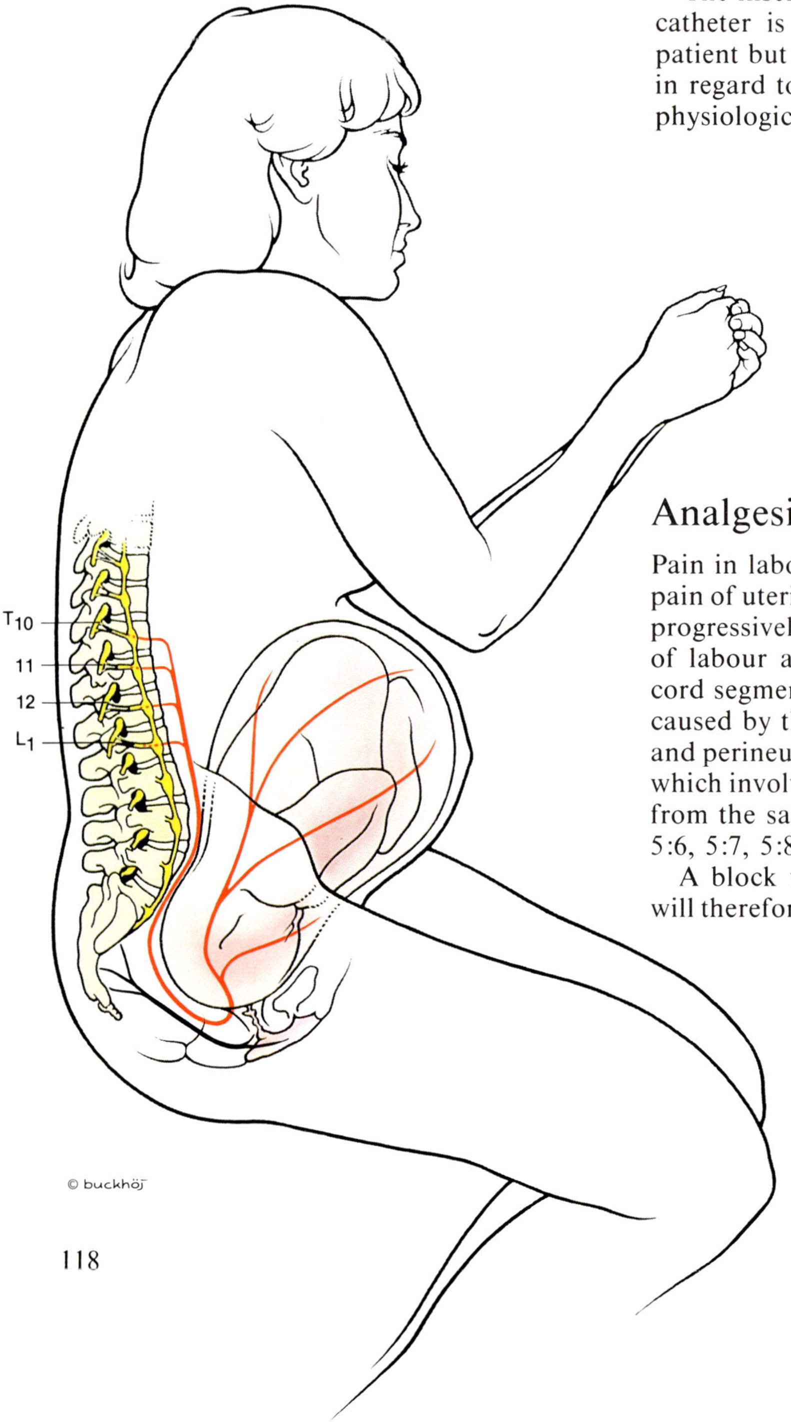

Fig. 5:6 Lateral view of afferent nerve pathways from the uterus and perineum.

Analgesia in labour

Pain in labour is of two kinds. Firstly, the pain of uterine contractions which becomes progressively more severe in the first stage of labour and is subserved by the spinal cord segments T_{10} - L_1. Secondly the pain caused by the stretching of the birth canal and perineum in the second stage of labour, which involves the pudendal nerve deriving from the sacral segments 2, 3 and 4 (Figs. 5:6, 5:7, 5:8).

A block which extends from T_{10} to S_5 will therefore give total relief of pain during the entire birth process. Because the pain of uterine contractions is mediated through sympathetic afferent nerve fibres, it is possible to achieve good analgesia with a block confined to the spinal segments T_{10} - L_1 in the first stage of labour. Such a block, moreover, does not require high concentrations of local anaesthetic. Some authorities therefore attempt to block these segments with a relatively high catheter inserted through the T_{12} - L_1 interspace and injection of a small volume (5-6 ml) of local anaesthetic. When the second stage of labour is reached, a larger volume (10 ml) of more concentrated solution is injected to block the S_{2-4} nerves and anaesthetise the perineum. This form of anaesthesia is referred to as segmental epidural block.

It has to be admitted, however, that most anaesthetists use the L_{2-3} or L_{3-4} interspace with a single catheter and obtain a block from T_{10} - S_5 throughout labour.

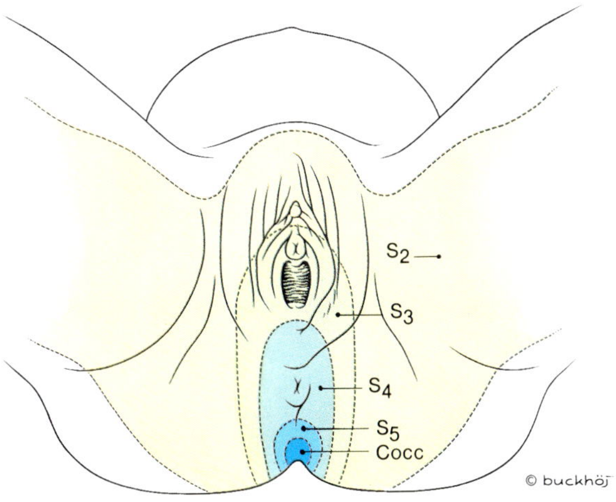

Fig. 5:8 Segmental nerve supply of the vulva and perineum.

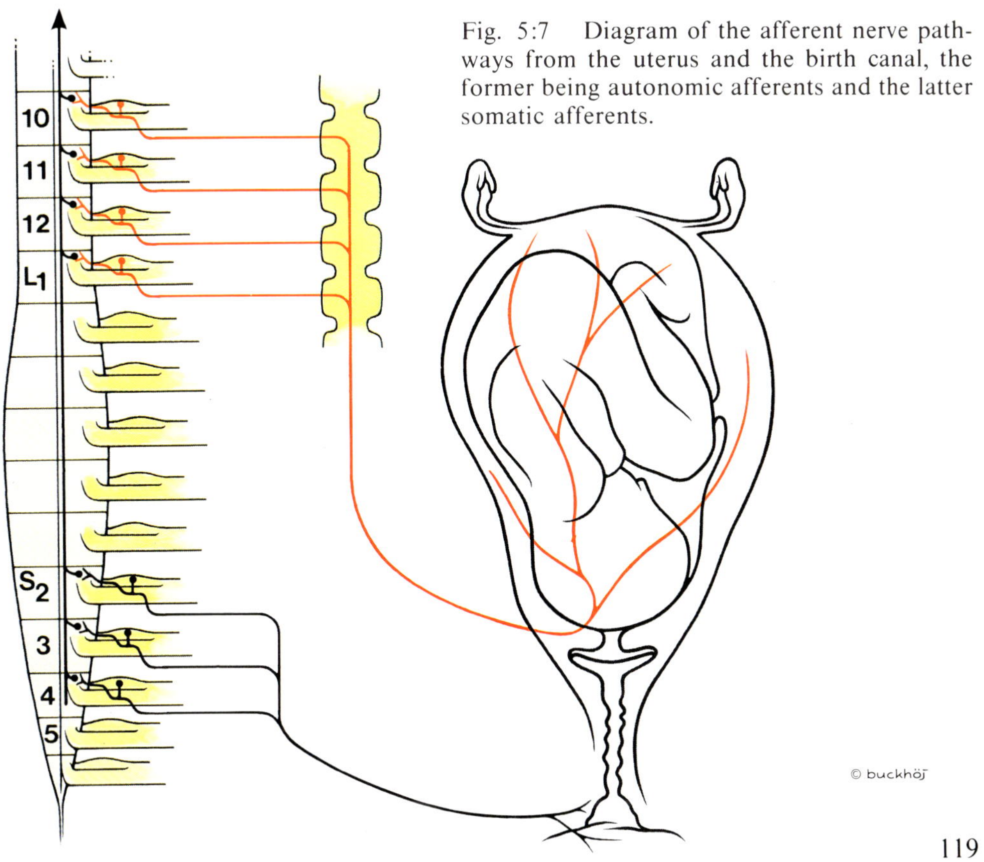

Fig. 5:7 Diagram of the afferent nerve pathways from the uterus and the birth canal, the former being autonomic afferents and the latter somatic afferents.

Drugs and dosage

The drug which has obtained the greatest popularity for epidural block in labour is bupivacaine. This is because it has a relatively long duration, thus decreasing the number of "top-up" injections, and seldom causes total paralysis of the legs, which many patients do not like.

Because of the limited block required and the fact that only sympathetic nerves are involved in the first stage, smaller doses and lower concentrations of local anaesthetics may be used. This has the advantage of reducing the amount of drug transferred to the foetus and the incidence, in the mother, of motor block in the lower limbs. However, the less drug that is given, the shorter is the duration of effect and therefore the more frequent are the top-ups.

Individual assessment of the patient is essential. The effect of the first main dose to be injected should be carefully monitored in regard to spread, effectiveness, motor block and any circulatory effects. From this knowledge, adjustments can be made in subsequent injections.

The following doses are recommended:

Test dose (see page 98): 3-4 ml of 0.5% bupivacaine with added epinephrine.

First main dose: 6-10 ml of 0.25% or 0.5% bupivacaine.

Subsequent top-ups: 6-12 ml of 0.25% or 0.5% bupivacaine according to the extent and degree of the nerve block produced by the first main dose.

Continous epidural infusion A continous infusion of dilute bupivicaine (0.125%) at a rate of 10-15 $ml.h^{-1}$ can be used. This greatly reduces the number of top-up injections that are required.

Top-ups in 2nd stage: 5-10 ml 0.5% bupivacaine.

Other drugs may be used in equivalent concentrations and the same volumes. For example, 2% lidocaine may be used for the test dose and first main dose. Its profound and relatively fast effect will allow an accurate assessment of the block and its shorter duration may be of value if the spread is unduly wide. For similar reasons, chloroprocaine 2%-3% may be used and has the advantage of low systemic toxicity and even shorter duration. Its abrupt cessation of action may cause contractions to become very painful before a top-up can take effect. The top-ups should be given as soon as the patient becomes aware of her contractions, i.e., before they become painful.

To ensure perineal anaesthesia in the second stage of labour, especially if episiotomy or forceps delivery are to be carried out, the higher concentrations of the local anaesthetics should be used (0.5% bupivacaine, 2% lidocaine).

Posture during injection

When injecting small quantities of local anaesthetic it is possible that gravity may affect the spread of the solution in the epidural space, leading to unilateral block. It is more likely, however, that unilateral block is due to the inability of small volumes to fill both sides of the epidural space. The position of the catheter tip is probably more important than gravity. With injections of 8 - 10 ml or more it is doubtful if gravity influences the spread. Injections are best given in the lateral position to avoid caval compression when supine.

Physiological effects of epidural block

In addition to the changes seen in non-pregnant patients (see p. 47) other effects may be seen in late pregnancy. After 24 weeks the pregnant uterus is a constant threat to the patency of the inferior vena cava and can exert pressure on the aorta when the patient lies supine. In late pregnancy, the supine position will occlude the vena cava in most women (Fig. 5:9), venous return being maintained by a collateral circulation via the azygos system of veins. If the venous return (and therefore the cardiac output) is reduced, there will be a reflex vasoconstriction to compensate and keep the arterial pressure normal. In such circumstances a sympathetic block will counteract this compensation and hypotension, sometimes profound, will result. Reductions of arterial pressure below 80 mmHg systolic are likely to cause serious underperfusion of the placenta.

This hypotension may also trigger a vasovagal attack with a further reduction in output and pressure (Fig. 5:10). A severe reduction in arterial pressure with bradycardia can occur very rapidly. The mother can become unconscious, and unless she is turned into the lateral position there is a danger of cerebral hypoxia (vide infra).

Fig. 5:9 Radiograph following injection of dye into both femoral veins during late pregnancy with the mother lying supine. Note total obstruction to inferior vena cava and collateral drainage through the paravertebral veins.

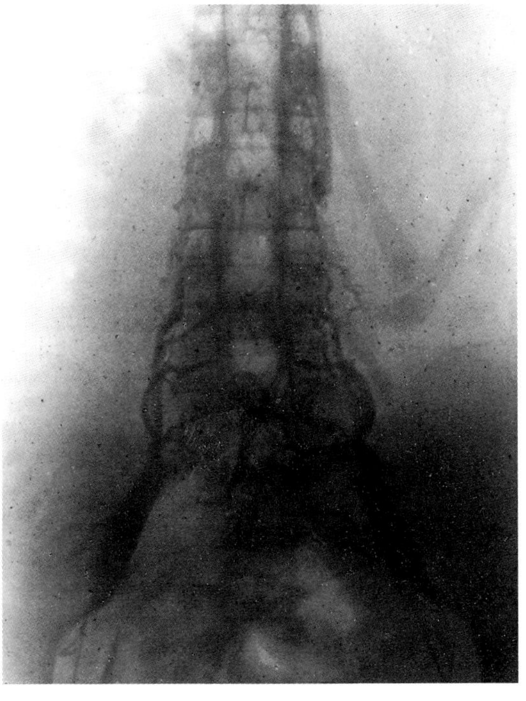

Fig. 5:10 Haemodynamic changes during late pregnancy consequent on turning from the lateral to the supine posture. Note that arterial pressure is maintained for a few minutes despite a reduction in cardiac output. The sudden development of a bradycardia and severe hypotension indicates a vaso-vagal attack.

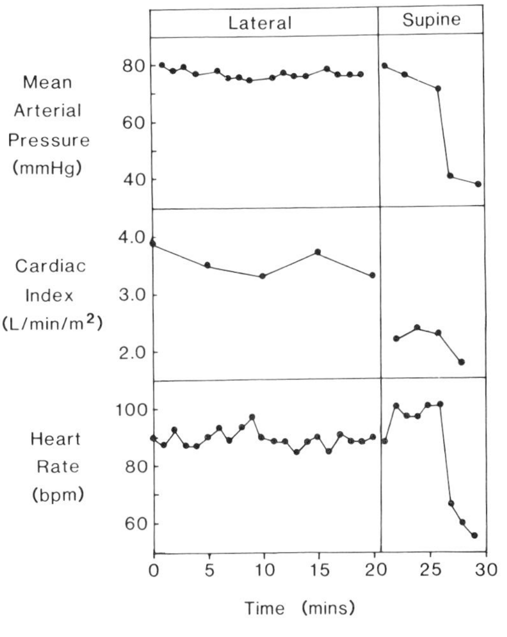

Owing to lack of voluntary expulsive efforts of the mother, the forceps rate is often increased when epidural blocks have been employed. The vast majority are outlet forceps and of no consequence to the neonate. A high spontaneous delivery rate can be achieved if the second stage is allowed to proceed for a sufficient time. Instrumental rotation of the foetal head, if necessary, can be performed with no further anaesthesia.

The nerve block will interfere with the perineal sphincters and micturition. The sensation of a full bladder is often not present, and catheterisation may be required.

Effects on maternal and foetal acid-base balance

The complete relief of pain in labour abolishes the bearing-down reflex in the second stage of labour. Thus much less physical work is required of the mother and the Valsalva effects of bearing-down are largely abolished. The result is a much smaller tendency towards acidosis, maternal and foetal, which is common even in uncomplicated labour. This is especially marked in the foetus, who is born significantly less acidotic than is the case with conventional analgesia (Fig. 5:11).

Pharmacological effects of epidural block

Local anaesthetics in sufficient dosage can affect uterine blood flow adversely. They can also cross the placenta, and equilibrium between mother and foetus in regard to the plasma concentrations of unbound drug is rapidly achieved with all drugs save chloroprocaine, which is destroyed in maternal plasma before very much of it can reach the foetus.

The use of epinephrine containing solutions in obstetrics remains controversial. It has been postulated that epinephrine will constrict uterine arteries and reduce placental blood flow, but this has not been confirmed by studies in which placental flow has been measured in humans. Moreover, if

Fig. 5:11 Changes in foetal base excess during labour. After Pearson and Davies. Reprinted from Principles and Practice of Obstetric Anaesthesia, J. S. Crawford.

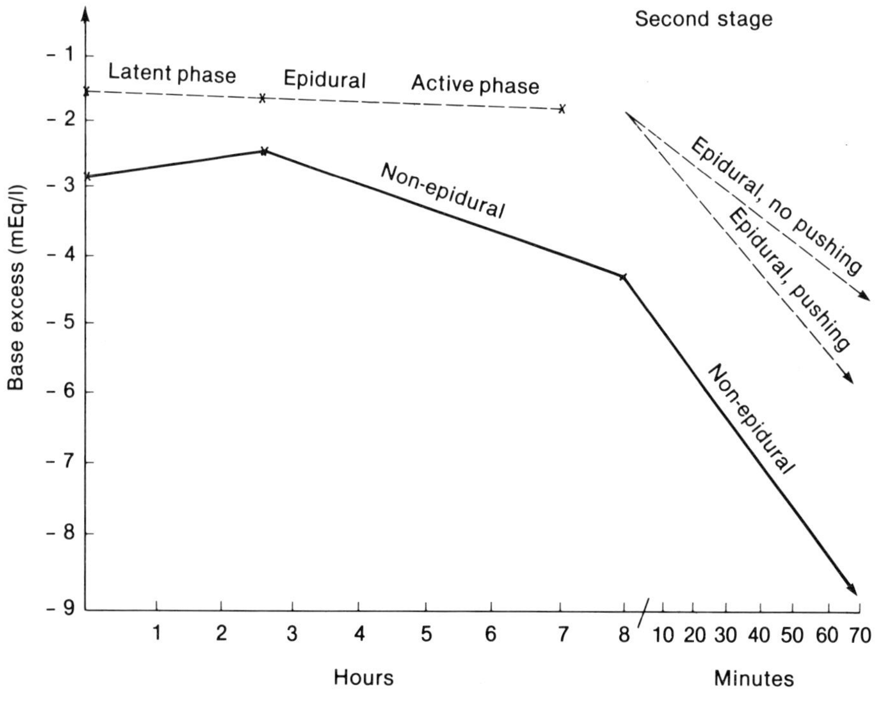

blood pressure is maintained, epidural block has been shown to cause a small but significant increase in placental flow. However, there is little need for epinephrine containing solutions during labour. Its use should be confined to test doses and possibly where a profound block is required for Caesarian section.

Plasma concentrations sufficient to have adverse effects will only be seen if the drugs are given intravenously by accident, and will be short-lived in the doses recommended above. The most likely effect will be transient toxicity related to the maternal central nervous system (numb tongue, lightheadedness, visual disturbances and muscular twitching, see p. 145).

Detailed neurobehavioural testing of neonates has shown minor deviations from normal in some (though not all) studies when epidural block has been used in labour. It is doubtful if they have any clinical significance and, contrary to the early views expressed, it is doubtful if the specific local anaesthetic used makes any difference to the incidence and severity of the observed abnormalities in neurobehavioural tests.

Complications

Hypotension

This may result from an unusually high sympathetic block (remembering the possibility of accidental subarachnoid injection) but is more usually due to the combination of inferior vena caval occlusion and sympathetic blockade, which may also trigger a vasovagal attack. The supine position is therefore best avoided. If it is adopted for any reason, the pulse should be felt throughout and the arterial pressure checked frequently. The pressure in any event should be measured every few minutes for 15 - 20 min after each epidural injection. If bradycardia develops then a vasovagal attack should be suspected. This can be accompanied by rapid profound hypotension and transient cardiac arrest with unconsciousness. The patient may complain of inability to breathe due to air hunger from the low cardiac output, but this may be misdiagnosed as respiratory failure due to a high subarachnoid block.

Hypotension can be largely prevented or modified by avoiding the supine position and by preloading the circulation with 500 - 1000 ml of electrolyte solution. If, however, the pressure falls below 80 mmHg ,a vasopressor (e.g., ephedrine 10 - 15 mg i.v.) should be given. Contrary to common opinion, atropine will seldom adequately counteract a vasovagal attack.

High blockade

While blocks reaching the upper thoracic segments are sometimes seen with volumes of 10 ml injected into the epidural space, the possibility of a subarachnoid or a subdural injection should be considered (see p. 161). The two important results of high blockade are hypotension and respiratory paralysis (indicating a motor block to C_3) The treatment is discussed on p. 162.

Inadequate block

Penetration of the spinal nerves by local anaesthetic may be inadequate if the weaker solutions are used or the volume injected is too small. This will result in the pain of uterine contractions being felt in the lower abdomen or groin (usually on one side only) and is due to inadequate blockade of L_1. This can invariably be corrected by re-injection with a more potent solution or a larger volume. This type of "missed segment" should not be confused with that seen with the first sacral nerve, which is difficult to block because of its size (see p. 39). As S_1 plays no role in the appreciation of pain in labour, inability to block it will be of no consequence.

Unilateral block which is sometimes seen is usually due to inadequate dosage.

Catheter problems

(see p. 167)

Headache

Spinal headache (see p. 163) is to be expected if a dural tap has occurred during the initial needling. The management is the same as with non-pregnant patients (see p. 164).

Episiotomy pain

This can be severe in patients after delivery when their epidural block has worn off. If the block has been very successful in relieving pain, the contrast when it disappears can be very great, especially as systemic analgesics will not have been given.

Neurological complications

Neurological complications are seen very occasionally, as with non-pregnant patients (see p. 165). However, the birth process, especially if it is instrumental, is also capable of causing nerve palsies and retention of urine. The vast majority of neurological complications are only temporary, lasting days or a few weeks.

Specific indications

• For abnormal presentations, especially the breech.

• For premature deliveries.

• When there is a high expectation of Caesarean or forceps delivery.

• In pre-eclamptic and hypertensive patients. A higher than usual block may be used as it helps to control the blood pressure. The absence of pain prevents increases in the arterial pressure during contractions.

Contra-indications

There are very few absolute contra-indications to the use of epidural block in labour. Relative contra-indications include:

a. Previous Caesarean section can lead to a ruptured uterine scar and if the epidural block is very dense, the pain of impending or actual rupture may be abolished. In such patients it is therefore better to use the lower concentrations of local anaesthetic e.g., 0.25% bupivacaine.

b. Infection in the skin at the site of injection would be a contra-indication, but infection widespread enough to prevent access through at least one intervertebral space must be extremely rare.

c. Coagulopathies are also rare in labouring women but may occur as part of disseminated intravascular coagulation caused by amniotic fluid embolus, severe pre-eclampsia or placental abruption.

d. Chronic neurological disease is not affected by epidural block and in the great majority of patients it presents no contra-indication.

e. Acute systemic infection with bacteraemia has been known to cause an epidural abscess, presumably by blood-borne bacteria colonising an epidural haematoma, though it has also been reported in a patient who did not receive an epidural block.

Caesarean section

Epidural block has become the anaesthetic method of choice in many centres for Caesarean sections. Its main advantage is that, unlike general anaesthesia, the mother can be kept conscious throughout. This has emotional attractions for many mothers, who wish to be awake at the birth of their baby. In addition it avoids the need to intubate the trachea and the risk of acid aspiration. Spinal anaesthesia shares these advantages and is generally faster in onset. However, with a catheter technique, epidural block is more controllable and may be prolonged for as long as is necessary.

For the foetus, regional anaesthesia obviates the need for central nervous system depressant drugs.

Caesarean section performed with epidural block presents certain problems:

Patient preparation. To avoid sedating the foetus, premedicant drugs are best avoided. This means that the epidural block must be as effective as possible. Thus dosage must be adequate and the necessary time for the block to develop must be taken. The patient should not be promised total analgesia as this is not obtainable in every case and even a minor amount of discomfort during surgery may cause a serious loss of confidence. The procedure should be explained as fully as possible. The presence of the patient's husband during the operation is frequently very helpful in maintaining her morale.

Drugs and dosage. Unlike analgesia in labour, a full nerve block is required and paralysis of the legs is to be expected. This is of little importance if it has been properly explained to the patient. The strongest solutions should be given, 2% lidocaine, 0.5% bupivacaine or 1.5% etidocaine. Epinephrine 1:200,000 will usually enhance the degree of nerve blockade and may be added. There is no evidence that it has an adverse effect on uterine blood flow. A volume of 15 - 20 ml is required to consistently achieve a block to the level of T_8. Some authorities like to inject smaller and repeated doses until a block of the decided height is obtained, often turning the patient from side to side. However, there is little evidence that posture affects the spread of solution in the epidural space, especially with high volume injections.

Onset of anaesthesia. It is desirable to have a short onset time in Caesarean section, especially if the section is for an urgent condition such as foetal distress. Some drugs commonly used, such as bupivacaine 0.5%, have a long onset time and 30 min. or more may have to be allowed before surgery can start. This may well be unacceptable. A more rapid onset can be achieved with lidocaine or etidocaine. Etidocaine is particularly quick, and the 1.5% solution with epinephrine will allow surgery to begin in most patients within 10-15 min of injection. However, it will also produce a profound motor block that will persist for several hours.

The first indication of a successful epidural injection is a feeling of warmth and tingling of the feet and lower limbs. Adequate analgesia for surgery will be indicated by the response of the patient to pinprick of the abdominal wall.

Hypotension. This will occur for the reasons given on p. 123. Inferior vena caval occlusion should be avoided, at least in part, by tilting to the left side. If, in spite of this, occlusion is suspected, the full lateral position should be adopted or the uterus displaced manually to the left. Preloading the patient with 500 - 1000 ml of crystalloid solution reduces the incidence of hypotension. If fainting occurs with bradycardia and nausea, a vasopressor will correct the situation rapidly. Ephedrine 5 - 15 mg i.v. will quickly increase both the heart rate and the arterial pressure. A phenylephrine drip can give more precise control of the arterial pressure.

Patient discomfort during surgery. Even apparently solid blocks sometimes fail to prevent visceral pain associated with stripping the bladder from the lower uterine segment, delivery of the neonate and stitching of the uterine incision. Before delivery of the baby, the mother should be encouraged to persevere in spite of discomfort. After delivery there is no contra-indication to giving additional medication. Clearly when pain is the main problem, analgesics are likely to be the most successful, and intravenous opioids (e.g., morphine 10 mg or fentanyl 100 μg) will invariably improve the situation considerably. Sedative drugs such as benzodiazepines are of little use if pain is the principal symptom and they should be reserved for occasions when agitation or nervousness is the main complaint.

If there is a total, or near total, failure to produce adequate analgesia, the patient may require a full general anaesthetic.

Oxytocics. These are given routinely after delivery. With conscious patients ergometrine is to be avoided as it is associated with a high incidence of nausea, and vomiting and can cause a considerable increase in arterial pressure in pre-eclamptic patients. Oxytocin 5 units as a bolus and 5 units added to the i.v. infusion, will ensure adequate uterine tone and has no emetic properties.

Epidural block in acute pain

The main indications for the use of epidural blockade in acute pain are relief of pain in labour (vide supra) and postoperative analgesia. In addition epidural block can be used to relieve painful states such as ureteric stone, acute pancreatitis and following trauma. Thoracic epidural block is now widely used for the relief of multiple fractured ribs. A catheter technique is used and top-ups or continuous infusions are given as indicated. With this method the need to ventilate patients is considerably reduced.

Postoperative analgesia

A nerve block which can provide anaesthesia for surgical operations can clearly provide analgesia in the postoperative period if the block is prolonged for a sufficient time. Because of the ease of inserting a catheter, epidural block can be prolonged indefinitely and is the most effective form of analgesia presently available in the postoperative period. In spite of this it is seldom employed for more than a few hours after surgery. The problem is essentially one of practicality. If the block is too extensive, there is an undesirable degree of both sympathetic and motor blockade. If it is confined to the few nerves supplying the area of the surgical wound, it is short in duration and requires frequent topping-up. Moreover, a narrow band of analgesia which renders the wound free of pain may not relieve other types of visceral pain such as that due to gas under the diaphragm.

To obtain the optimal benefit from epidural block it is therefore necessary to:

- Limit the block to the area of the wound while affecting as few motor and sympathetic nerves as possible.

• Provide alternative analgesia such as intramuscular opioid for any pain arising outside the blocked area.

A narrow band of analgesia can be achieved by siting the catheter at or near the centre of the area to be blocked, e.g., between T_{11} and T_{12} for lower abdominal surgery or T_8 and T_9 for upper abdominal surgery.

With thoracic operations the level of the incision will govern the site of the catheter while for hip operations the lumbar region will suffice.

Assuming the operation has been performed under epidural block, this should be maintained by a top-up injection of 6-10 ml of 0.5% bupivacaine at the end of surgery. Ideally the block should not be allowed to wear off. It can be maintained by the frequent injection of small volumes of 0.5% bupivacaine (e.g., 4-6 ml every hour) or by the continuous infusion of dilute bupivacaine (e.g. 20 ml. hour^{-1} of 0.1% or 15 ml. hour^{-1} of 0.125%). Frequent small bolus injections can be made with an electronically controlled pump while continuous infusions need a simple infusion pump.

Management

Patients with prolonged epidural block must be carefully monitored, especially in regard to their cardiovascular status. Arterial pressure and heart rate should be measured frequently, particularly following bolus injections.

Fluid balance should be well maintained to counteract the vasodilation produced by the sympathetic blockade. Urine output should be recorded. The level of the block should be checked occasionally, together with the ability to move the lower limbs, and note should be made if the degree of motor block appears to be increasing.

Pressure points (especially the heels) should be protected and the patient moved from time to time.

The appearance of pain, its degree and location, should be recorded.

Patients can lose considerable heat during surgery under epidural block and may complain of feeling cold and shivering postoperatively. An electric blanket is useful in preventing or treating this.

Complications

Hypotension

Hypotension is the most feared complication though it is easy to prevent and to treat. Systolic pressures in the region of 80-100 mmHg are common in the first few hours following surgery, regardless of the anaesthetic and postoperative analgesia given. In the vast majority of patients this degree of hypotension is quite acceptable provided the patient is not sitting upright. A liberal policy with intravenous fluids will usually prevent hypotension, and the rapid infusion of 250-500 ml of electrolyte solution will raise the arterial pressure if it decreases unduly. As a temporary measure, the foot of the bed should be raised while fluids are being given rapidly to correct hypotension.

Finally, vasopressors are occasionally necessary. To obtain a prolonged effect the intramuscular route is indicated. Ephedrine 15-30 mg is very suitable and effective, and may be used prophylactically. Patients with hypotension which either recurs or does not respond to simple treatment should be suspected of bleeding and appropriate investigation and therapy initiated.

Inadequate analgesia

Inadequate analgesia may be due to insufficient dosage of local anaesthetic or to the appearance of visceral or referred pain. In the former case the block should be reinforced with a bolus injection of 0.5% bupivacaine while the dosage of the continuous or intermittent injections should be increased. Unilateral block sometimes occurs and may be corrected by withdrawal of the catheter by a few millimetres or by increasing the dose of local anaesthetic.

If pain is thought to be visceral in type, a dose of opioid equivalent to 10 mg morphine may be given intramuscularly. This is of particular value during the night, as the sedative effects of these drugs will assist the patient in sleeping. Visceral pain is seldom as severe as the pain which comes from the surgical wound and indeed is often only appreciated when the wound pain is completely relieved. It will almost always respond to modest doses of opioid and respiratory depression will not be a problem.

Urinary retention

Urinary retention will occur if the block extends into the sacral area, and catheterisation will be necessary. However, many patients can be treated without blocking the sacral roots and can empty their bladders spontaneously.

Motor blockade

Motor blockade of the lower limbs is often disliked by the patient and should be avoided if possible. However, the fear that it may lead to deep venous thrombosis need not be entertained as the sympathetic blockade ensures an increase in lower limb blood flow.

Epidural opioids for postoperative pain are discussed on p. 77.

Epidural block in chronic pain

In recent years the use of nerve blocks in treating chronic pain has declined somewhat, particularly in pain not associated with malignant disease.

However, several conditions can be treated with epidural blockade. The most common of these are:

Chronic lower back pain

The injection of local anaesthetic will of course relieve the pain for the duration of its action. The addition of a long-acting corticosteroid, however, will reduce any inflammatory changes that are present and can often produce prolonged improvement.

Chronic non-malignant pain

It is possible to insert an epidural catheter and leave it in situ for days or weeks. Frequent top-ups are made to see if the vicious circle of inappropriate pain can be broken.

Chronic malignant pain

Again, a catheter can be inserted into the epidural space and left for the duration of the patient's life. It is helpful to leave several inches of the catheter subcutaneously so that it emerges from the side or front of the patient rather than the back (Fig. 5:12). The patient or the relatives can be instructed in terms of appropriate dose and frequency of administration of either local anaesthetic or opioid. A bacterial filter will help protect against infection, and should be used routinely.

Although phenol injections which cause more permanent nerve block are more commonly used in the subarachnoid space, there is a growing use of epidural phenol injections for relieving malignant pain. Phenol 6%-8% is used in small (1 - 2 ml) aliquots until the desired blockade is obtained.

Fig. 5:12 a. b. and c. For prolonged epidural pain therapy a catheter can be tunnelled subcutaneously to appear in the lateral or anterior part of the trunk rather than the back. a. After placing the epidural catheter a large curved needle is inserted close to the catheter and tunnelling transversely across the trunk. b. After removing the blue plastic guard the catheter is threaded through the needle and leaves the trunk through the skin of the abdominal wall. c. The needle is removed leaving the catheter protruding from the abdominal wall. By pulling gently, the excess catheter at the back disappears into the subcutaneous tissue.
Photographs by Dr N.H. Gordon.

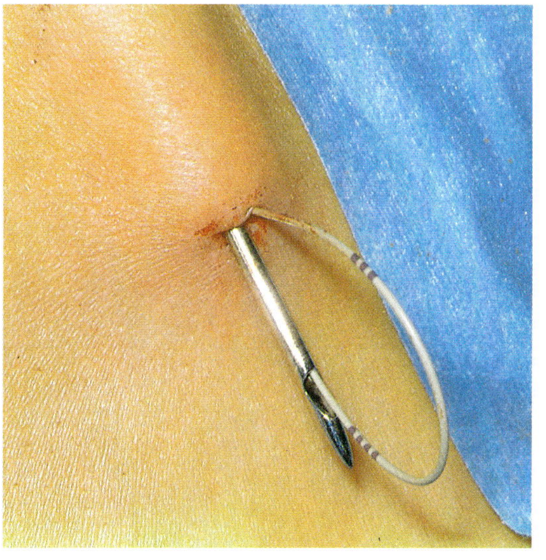

Fig. 5:12a

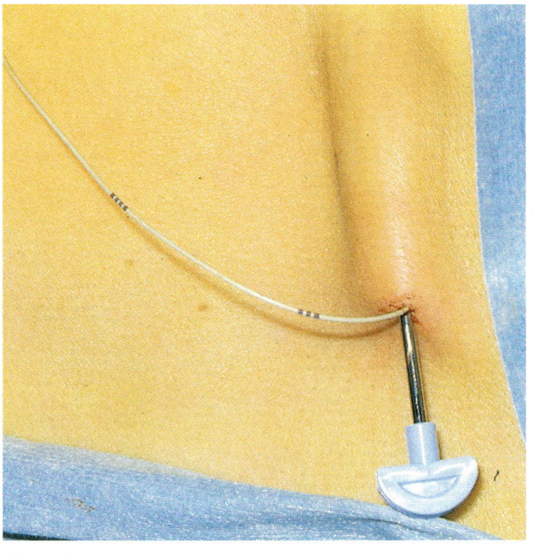

Fig. 5:12b

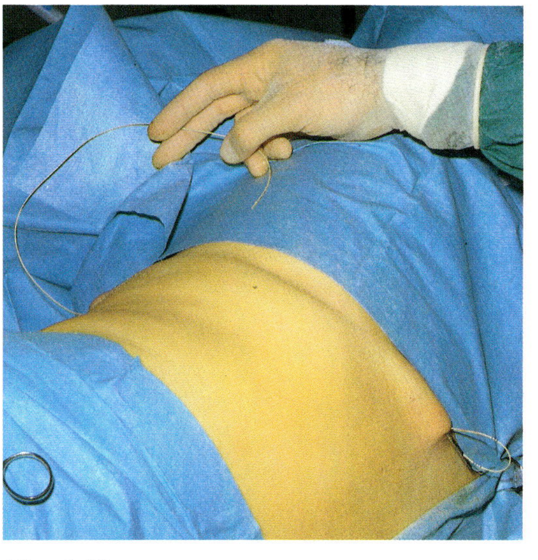

Fig. 5:12c

References & Bibliography

Aitkenhead, A.R., Wishart, H.Y. and Peebles-Brown, D.A. (1978). High spinal nerve block for large bowel anastomosis. Brit. J. Anaesth. 50, 177.

Crawford, J.S. (1978). Principles and Practice of Obstetric Anaesthesia. Blackwell, Oxford.

Griffiths, H.W.C. & Gilles, J. (1948). Thoraco - lumbar splanchnicectomy and sympathectomy: Anaesthetic procedure. Anaesthesia 3, 134.

Hollmen, A.I., Jouppila, R. Jouppila, P., Koivula, A. and Vierola, H. (1982). Effect of extradural analgesia using bupivacaine and 2-chloroprocaine on intervillous blood flow during normal labour. Brit. J. Anaesth. 54, 837.

Keith, I. (1977). Anaesthesia and blood loss in total hip replacement. Anaesthesia 32, 444.

Kerr, M.G., Scott, D.B. and Samuel, E. (1964). Studies of the inferior vena cava in late pregnancy. Br. Med. J.I., 532.

Lees, M.M., Kerr, M.G., Scott, D.B. and Taylor, S.H. (1967). Circulatory effects of the supine position in late pregnancy. Clin. Sci. 32, 453.

Modig, J. (1982). Thromboembolism and blood loss: Continuous epidural block versus general anesthesia with controlled ventilation. Regional Anesthesia. 7 (suppl.), 584.

Moir, D.D. (1976). Obstetric Anaesthesia and Analgesia. Bailliere Tindall, London.

Moroshima, H.O., Pedersen, H., Finster, M., Sakuma, K., Bruce, S.L., Gutsche, B.B, Stark, R.I. and Covino, B.G. (1981). Toxicity of lidocaine in adult, newborn and fetal sheep. Anesthesiology 61, 57.

Pearson, J.F. and Davies, P. (1974). The effect of continous lumbar epidural analgesia upon fetal acid-base status during the first stage of labour. J. Obstet. Gynaecol. Br. Commonw. 81, 971.

Pearson, J.F. & Davies, P. (1974). The effect of continous epidural analgesia upon fetal acid-base status in the second stage of labour. J. Obstet, Gynaecol. Br. Commonw. 81, 975.

Scott, D.B., Thorn, J. and Schweitzer, S.A. (1982). Epidural block for postoperative pain relief. Regional Anesthesia 7, 135.

Scott, D.B. (1983). Practical Regional Anaesthesia. Eds. Henderson J.J. and Nimmo, W.S. Blackwell, Edinburgh p. 229.

Thorud, T., Lund, I. and Holme, I. (1975). The effect of anesthesia on intraoperative and postoperative bleeding during abdominal proctatectomies. Acta Anaesthesiol. Scand. 57 [Suppl.]:83.

6. Complications of epidural anaesthesia

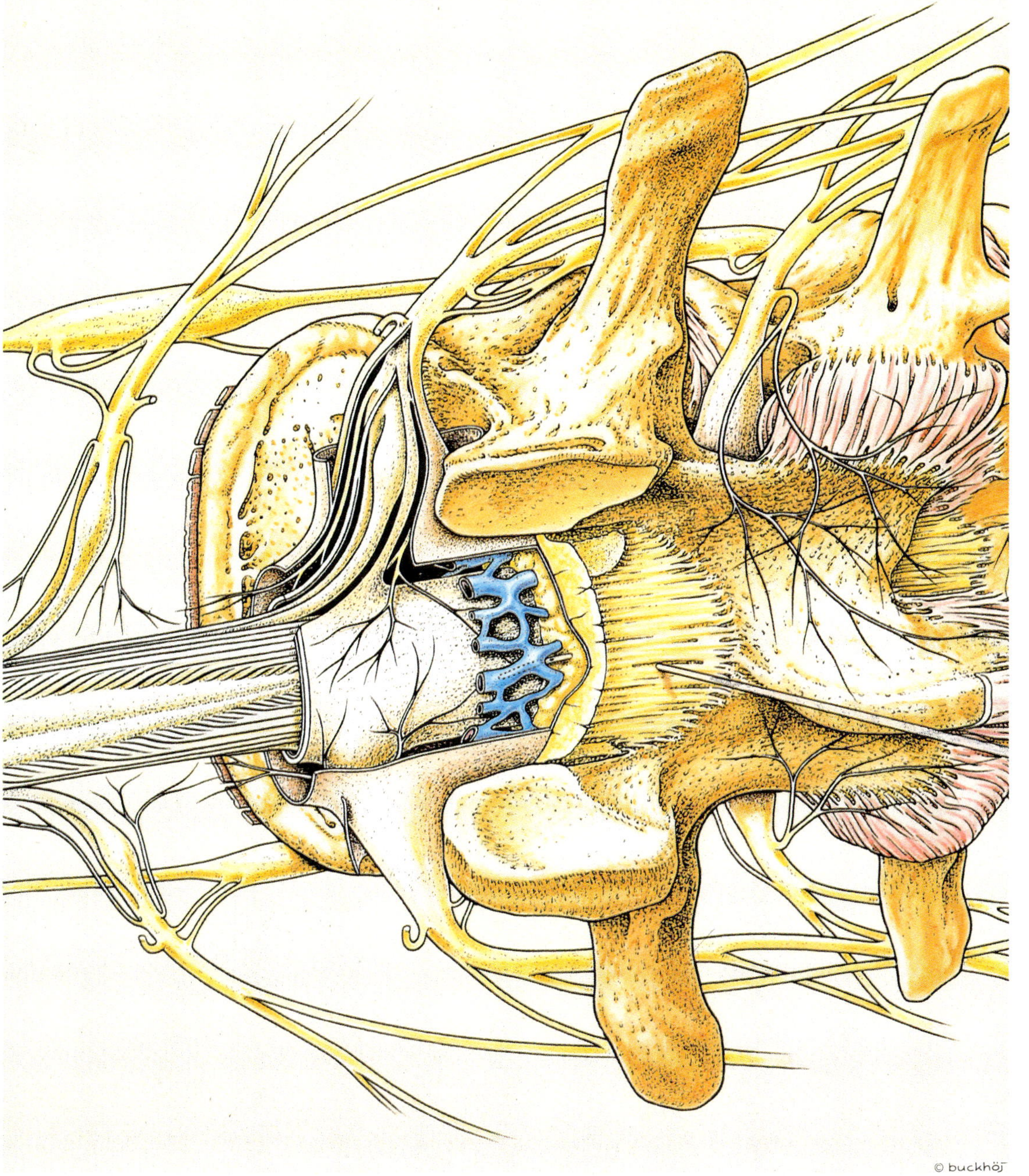

Drug related complications

Pharmacokinetic considerations

Relatively large doses of local anaesthetic agents are required in order to achieve adequate sensory anaesthesia for surgery following epidural administration. In addition, the epidural space contains numerous venous plexuses which may be penetrated by an epidural needle or catheter, leading

Fig. 6:1 Diagram of the epidural space showing the venous plexuses. Upper curves show local anaesthetic plasma levels following epidural administration (a) and accidental intravascular administration (b).

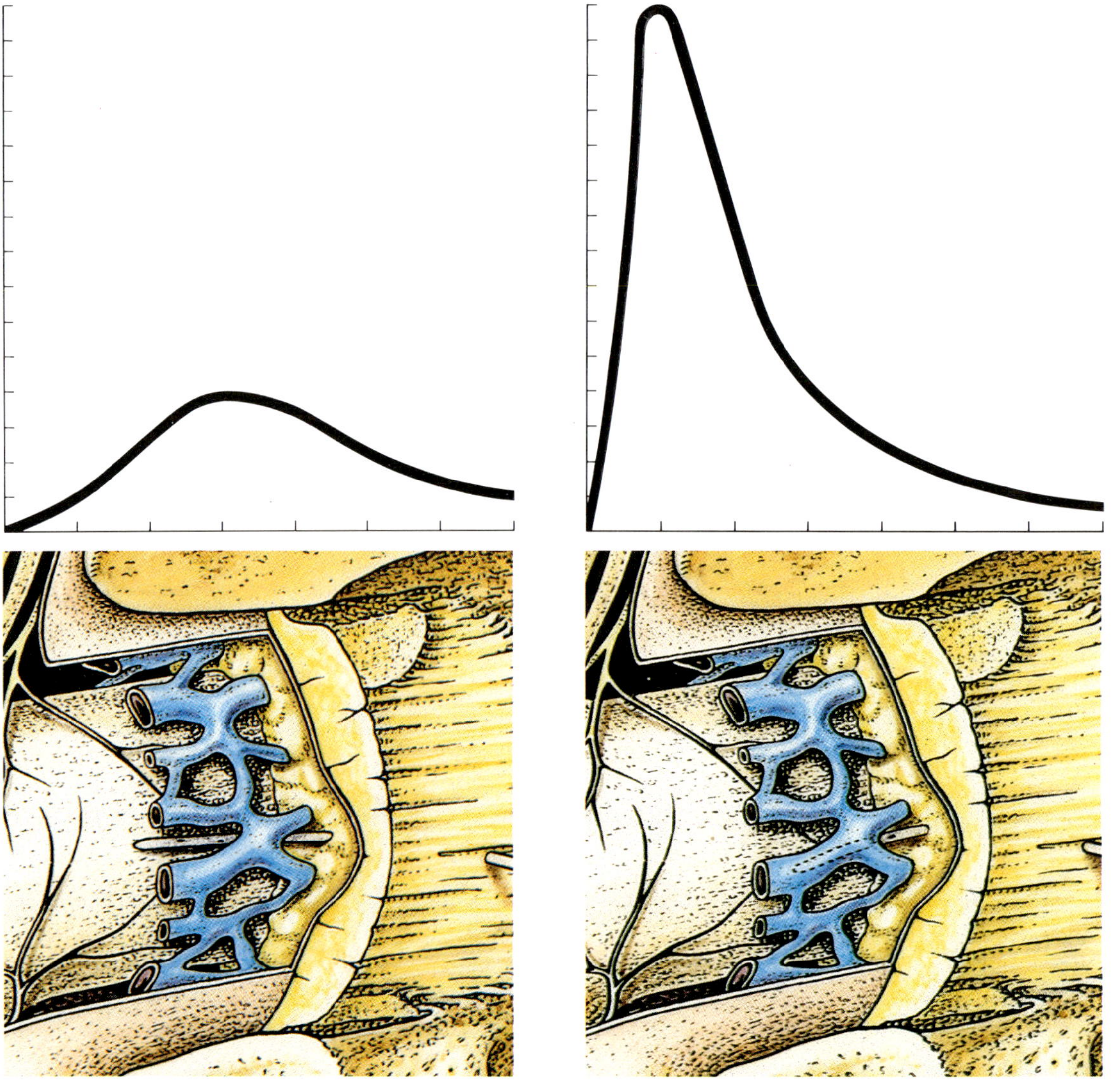

© buckhöj © buckhöj

to the accidental intravascular administration of local anaesthetic agents (Fig. 6:1a and b). As a result, toxicity may occur due either to the administration of an excessive amount of drug extravascularly or to accidental intravascular injection. The blood and tissue levels of local anaesthetic agents associated with systemic toxic reactions are determined by the rate of absorption, tissue redistribution, metabolism and excretion of the anaesthetic compound. Thus, a knowledge of the pharmacokinetic properties of local anaesthetic agents is of particular importance in the performance of epidural blockade in order to prevent the occurrence of adverse reactions.

It should be remembered that much higher plasma levels will occur with intravenous injection than by normal absorption. The rate of intravenous injection greatly affects the plasma level achieved, fast injections giving higher levels than slow injections (Fig. 6:2).

Fig 6:2 Relationship between arterial concentration of local anaesthetic following rapid I.V., slow I.V., and epidural administration.

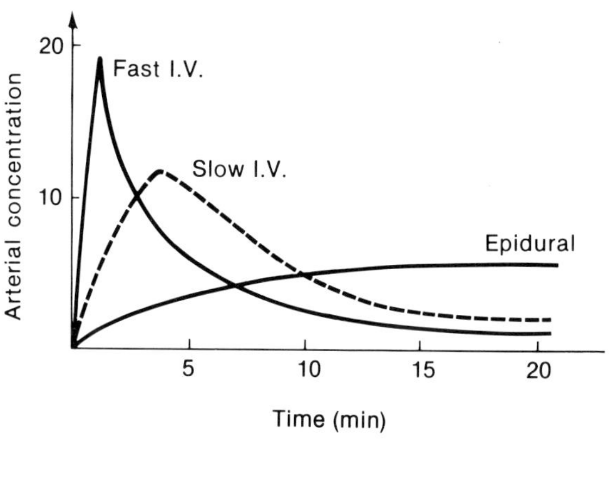

Absorption

The systemic absorption and potential toxicity of local anaesthetic agents are related to the site of injection, dosage, addition of a vasoconstrictor agent and the pharmacological profile of the agent itself. The rate of absorption of local anaesthetics varies considerably, depending on the vascularity of the injection site. For example, significantly higher plasma levels of local anaesthetics are achieved during intercostal blocks as compared with brachial plexus blockade. With regard to the epidural administration of local anaesthetics, little difference in the rate of absorption is seen following cervical, thoracic or lumbar epidural injections (Fig. 6:3). However, with caudal injections, mean peak venous plasma levels are significantly higher than those following other epidural injections. This may reflect exposure to a larger vascular surface area in the caudal canal.

Fig. 6:3 Relationship between venous plasma levels of lidocaine and administration of the same dose into various sites in the epidural space.

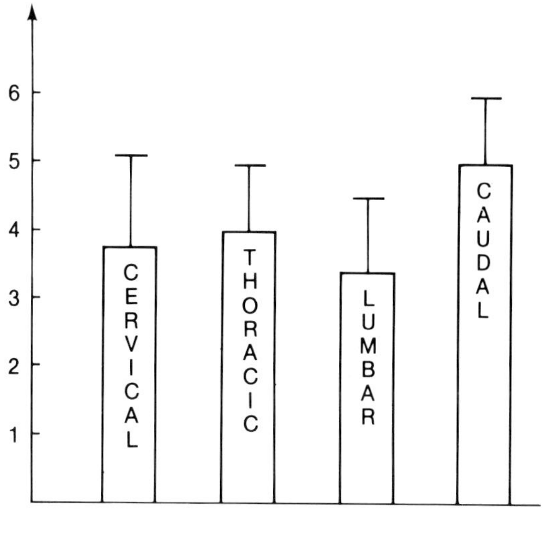

Blood levels of local anaesthetic agents are related to the total dose of drug administered. For most agents a linear relationship exists between the amount of drug administered and the resultant peak blood level (Fig. 6:4). For example, the mean venous blood level of lidocaine increased from approximately 1.5 μg.ml^{-1} to 4 μg.ml^{-1} as the total dose administered into the lumbar epidural space was increased from 200 to 600 mg. For certain local anaesthetics, such as bupivacaine and etidocaine, a nonlinear relationship has been observed between the total dose administered and the peak venous blood level. This may be due to the high lipid solubility of bupivacaine and etidocaine, which results in sequestration of these drugs in epidural fat, such that the rate of systemic absorption is less when relatively small doses are used. However, when large doses are administered, lipid depots may be saturated so that more free drug is available for absorption.

The peak blood level achieved following epidural blockade is a function of the dose in milligrams and does not appear to be related to either the concentration or volume of the local anaesthetic solution employed. No significant differences in the venous plasma levels of different local anaesthetics have been observed following the lumbar epidural administration of these agents at varying volumes and concentrations if the total dose was the same (Fig. 6:5) Generally speaking, a peak venous plasma level of approximately 1 μg.ml^{-1} will be achieved for every 100 mg lidocaine administered into the lumbar epidural space. Since venous plasma levels of 5 μg.ml^{-1} or less of lidocaine are rarely associated with toxic symptoms, the maximum single dose of lidocaine that can be safely administered epidurally is approximately 500 mg.

Many local anaesthetic solutions contain a vasoconstrictor agent, usually epinephrine in a concentration of 5 μg.ml^{-1} (1:200,000). The rationale for adding a vasoconstrictor agent is to prolong the duration by increasing neuronal uptake of the

Fig. 6:4 Relationship between the peak venous plasma level of various local anaesthetics and the dose administered epidurally.

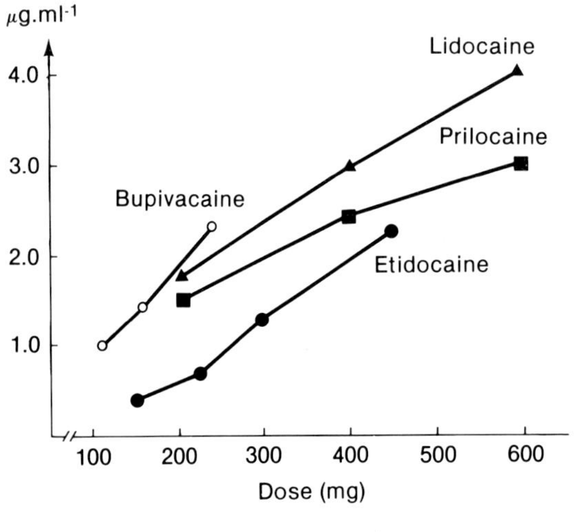

Fig. 6:5 Relationship between venous plasma levels of various local anaesthetics following epidural administration of varying volumes and concentrations.

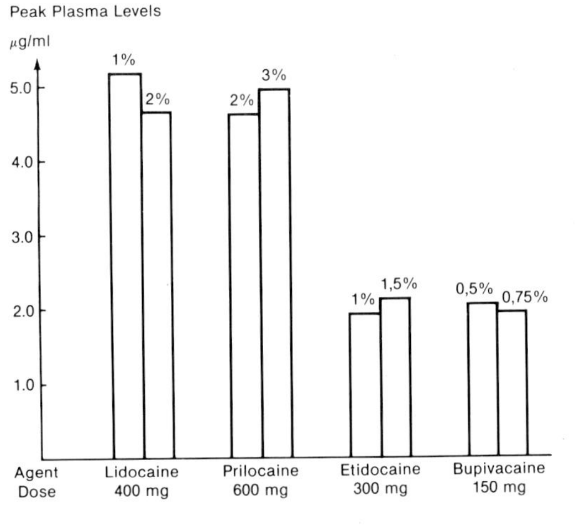

local anaesthetic and to reduce toxicity by decreasing the rate of absorption from the epidural space. A concentration of 5 μg.ml^{-1} of epinephrine appears to be optimal in terms of reducing the rate of absorption of local anaesthetic agents such as lidocaine and mepivacaine from the lumbar epidural space. The use of 12.5 μg.ml^{-1} (1:80,000) was not associated with a significantly greater reduction in the peak blood level. Other vasoconstrictor agents such as phenylephrine and norepinephrine have been employed in combination with local anaesthetic drugs. However, neither drug appears to be as effective as epinephrine 1:200,000 (Fig. 6:6).

The vascular uptake from the epidural space of agents such as prilocaine, bupivacaine and etidocaine appears to be less influenced by the addition of a vasoconstrictor than is the uptake of lidocaine and mepivacaine (Fig. 6:7). The decreased efficacy of epinephrine added to prilocaine solutions may be attributable to the extremely rapid rate of tissue redistribution of prilocaine. In addition, prilocaine may exert less of a vasodilator effect than lidocaine. The diminished influence of epinephrine on the absorption of bupivacaine and etidocaine may be related in part to the high lipid solubility of these two agents, which results in a significant uptake by epidural adipose tissue. In addition, the greater vasodilating potential of bupivacaine and etidocaine as compared with lidocaine may tend to counteract the vasoconstrictor effect of epinephrine.

Fig. 6:6 Effect of phenylephrine and epinephrine on the absorption of lidocaine from the epidural space.

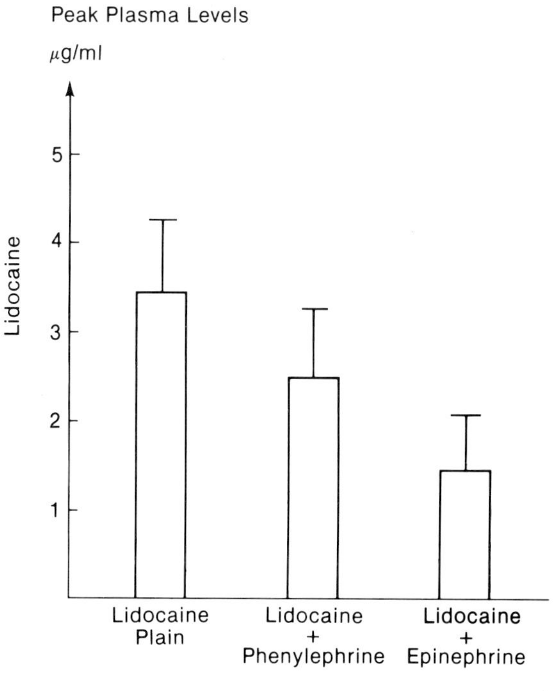

Fig. 6:7 Effect of epinephrine on the absorption of various local anaesthetics following administration into the epidural space.

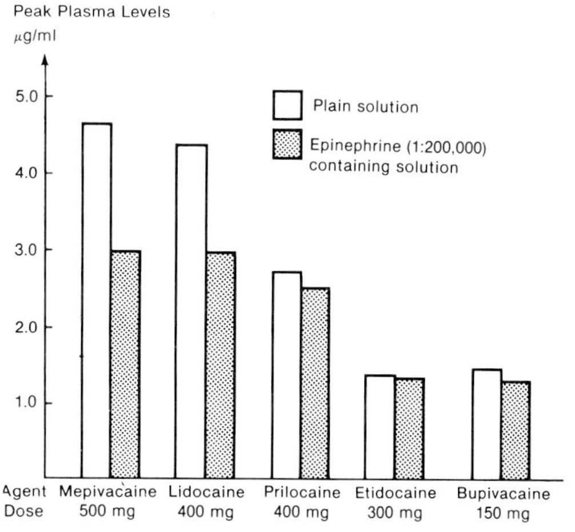

The variation in the rate of absorption of various local anaesthetics following administration into the epidural space is due also to the pharmacological properties of the various agents themselves. For example, a comparison of agents of equivalent anaesthetic potency reveals that lidocaine and mepivacaine show similar peak venous plasma levels following lumbar epidural administration. However, prilocaine plasma levels are significantly lower at all time periods (Fig. 6:8). This difference may reflect the greater vasodilator activity of mepivacaine and lidocaine, but more important is the larger distribution volume and the rapid rate of elimination of prilocaine. Among the more potent agents, etidocaine plasma levels are significantly lower than those of bupivacaine if equal doses of both agents are administered epidurally. This may be related in part to the greater lipid solubility, the larger distribution volume and the more rapid rate of elimination of etidocaine. The lower blood level of etidocaine has practical clinical implications. Although 1.0%-1.5% etidocaine is required to yield a degree of analgesia similar to that provided by 0.5%-0.75% bupivacaine, no difference in blood levels or potential toxicity exists between the two agents following lumbar epidural administration.

Fig. 6:8 Venous plasma levels of lidocaine and prilocaine following epidural administration.

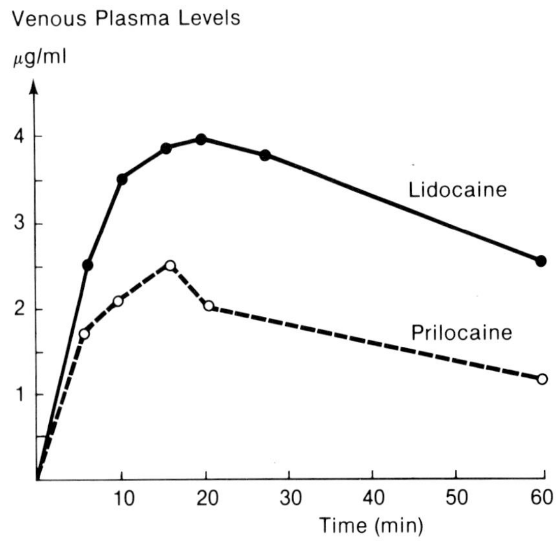

Fig. 6:9 The various sites of distribution.

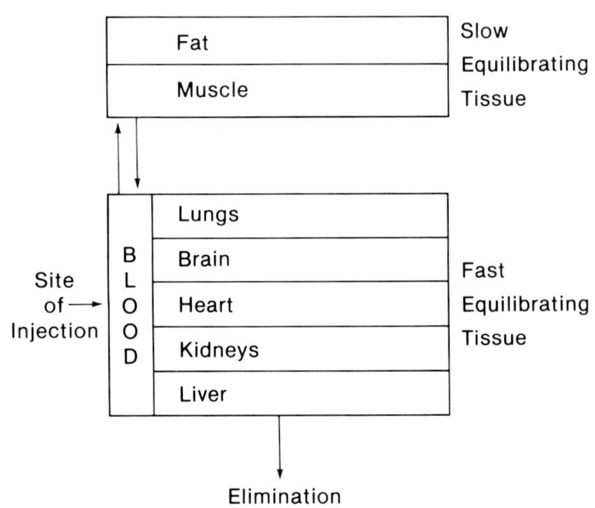

Distribution

Local anaesthetic agents are distributed from the central vascular compartment throughout total body water. The rate of disappearance of local anaesthetic drugs from blood, the volume of distribution and the relative uptake by various tissues are related to the physicochemical properties of the specific agents. The distribution of local anaesthetic agents can be described by a two compartment model (Fig. 6:9). The initial rapid phase of disappearance from blood (the alpha or distribution phase) is believed to be related to the uptake of these agents by rapidly equilibrating tissues, i.e., tissues which have a high vascular perfusion. The slower or secondary phase of disappearance from blood is mainly a function of distribution to slowly equilibrating tissues together with the metabolism and elimination of the compounds (elimination or beta phase). A comparison of the three amino amides of similar anaesthetic potency and duration of action, i.e., lidocaine, mepivacaine and prilocaine, reveals that prilocaine is redistributed more rapidly from blood to tissues than are lidocaine and mepivacaine. The rate of tissue redistribution for lidocaine and mepivacaine appears to be similar. Differences also exist between bupivacaine and etidocaine, the latter having a more rapid rate of tissue redistribution than bupivacaine (Table 6:1).

Table 6:1
Pharmacokinetic Properties of Various Amide Local Anaesthetics

Agent	T/2 (min)	T/2 (min)	V_D $_{SS}$(L)	T/2 Y (hours)	Cl (l/min)
Prilocaine	0.5	5.0	261	1.5	2.84
Lidocaine	1.0	9.6	91	1.6	0.95
Mepivacaine	0.7	7.2	84	1.9	0.78
Bupivacaine	2.7	28.0	72	3.5	0.47
Etidocaine	2.2	19.0	133	2.6	1.22

Although local anaesthetic agents are distributed throughout all body tissues, the relative uptake by different tissues varies with regard to rate of uptake and total tissue concentration. In general, the more highly perfused organs show higher concentrations of drug than the less perfused organs. Thus, the greatest concentration is found in lung and kidney which are highly vascularised organs (Fig. 6:10). However, the highest percentage of an injected dose of a local anaesthetic agent occurs in skeletal muscle. Although this tissue does not show any particular affinity for local anaesthetics, the large mass of skeletal muscle makes it the largest reservoir for a local anaesthetic agent. In the initial phase of tissue redistribution, the lung, through which all the absorbed drug must pass, appears to play a predominant role in the removal of local anaesthetics from the vascular compartment. Differences in the rate of

Fig. 6:10 Bar graph showing uptake of prilocaine by various organs.

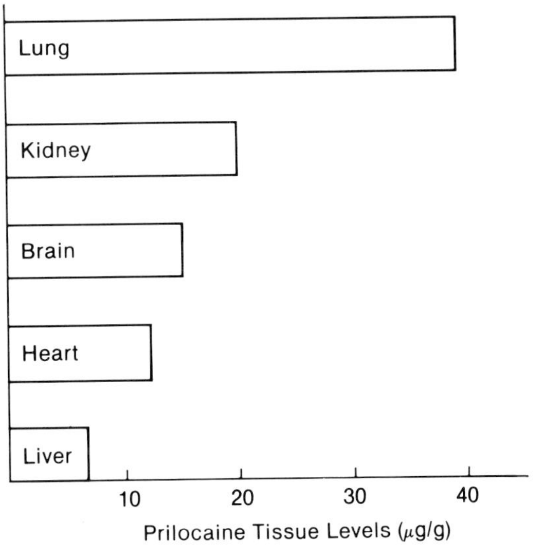

uptake by the lung may exist between various agents based on differences in plasma protein binding and lipid solubility (Fig. 6:11).

Local anaesthetics are bound primarily to αl-acid glycoproteins in plasma. Differences in the degree of plasma protein binding of the various agents will influence in part their rates of tissue distribution. For example, a correlation exists between the degree of plasma protein binding and the plasma/erythrocyte (P/E) ratio of the different agents. Bupivacaine and etidocaine are approximately 95% bound to plasma proteins and demonstrate a P/E ratio of approximately 8. On the other hand, prilocaine, which has a P/E ratio of 0.88, is only 55% bound to plasma proteins. Lidocaine and mepivacaine are intermediate in terms of plasma protein binding (64%-77%), and demonstrate P/E ratios of 1.34-2.6.

The ratio of placental transfer of local anaesthetic agents is also correlated with the degree of plasma protein binding (Fig. 6:12). Although equilibrium between maternal and umbilical venous blood will be quickly reached in regard to free unbound drug, the foetal/maternal (F/M) ratio varies with each drug if one considers the total (bound and unbound) drug concentration. This is because the degree of binding to foetal plasma proteins is less than the binding to maternal plasma proteins. Bupivacaine and etidocaine show F/M values of 0.14 to 0.44 and are also the agents which are most highly protein bound in maternal blood. Prilocaine shows the highest F/M ratio (1.0-1.8) and is the least protein bound

Fig. 6:11 Graph showing uptake of prilocaine and lidocaine by lung tissue.

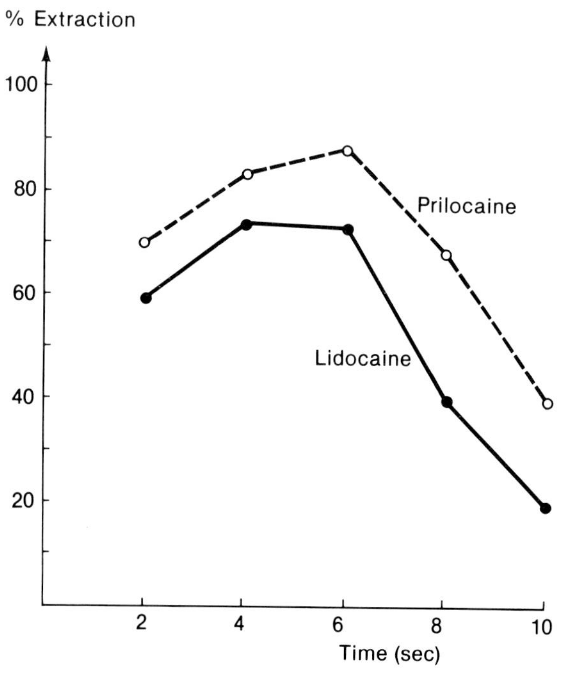

Fig. 6:12 Relationship between foetal-maternal (F/M) ratio and plasma protein binding of various local anaesthetics.

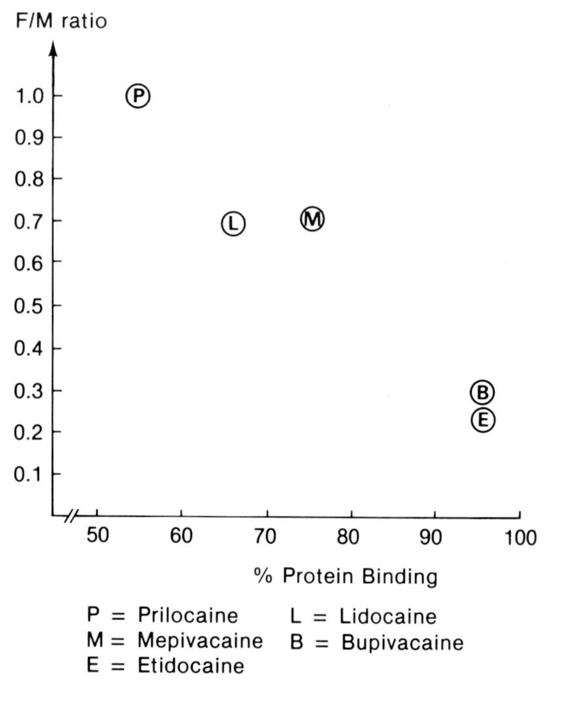

agent. Lidocaine and mepivacaine have F/M ratios of 0.52-0.71, which correlates with their plasma protein binding values of 64% -77%. A low F/M ratio does not indicate that less drug is reaching the foetus; in fact foetal tissue levels of all local anaesthetics are similar since tissue uptake is dependent upon the free drug concentration (Table 6:2).

The uptake of local anaesthetics by poorly perfused tissues such as skeletal muscle and fat is related both to their degree of plasma protein binding and their lipid solubility. For example, simultaneous measurements of local anaesthetic levels in the brachial artery and the antecubital vein show a venous-arterial blood concentration ratio of 0.73 for lidocaine and 0.47 for prilocaine. Thus, the rate of diffusion into muscle is considerably faster for prilocaine than for lidocaine, which is probably due to the lower plasma protein binding of prilocaine. On the other hand, tissue distribution studies of bupivacaine and etidocaine have shown that etidocaine is taken up to a considerably greater extent by peripheral fat than is bupivacaine. Since the degree of plasma protein binding of these two agents is similar, this difference in uptake by peripheral fat depots appears to be related to the greater lipid solubility of etidocaine.

Table 6:2
Mean (SE) Tissue/Blood Concentration Ratios in Guinea Pig Foetus

	Bupivacaine	Lidocaine
Brain	2.4 ± 0.5	2.0 ± 0.4
Heart	3.3 ± 0.7	1.8 ± 0.4
Lungs	3.3 ± 0.1*	2.0 ± 0.4
Liver	1.9 ± 0.8	0.5 ± 0.1
Kidneys	4.8 ± 0.4	4.0 ± 0.5
Adrenals	5.5 ± 0.7*	2.9 ± 0.5

* Significantly Different from Lidocaine

Metabolism and excretion of local anaesthetic agents

Metabolism of local anaesthetic agents varies according to their chemical structure. The amino ester or procaine-like drugs undergo hydrolysis in plasma by the enzyme pseudocholinesterase. The rate of hydrolysis varies markedly between agents in the same class. Chloroprocaine is hydrolysed at a rate of 4.7 $\mu mol.ml.h^{-1}$ compared with rates of 1.1 $\mu mol.ml.h^{-1}$ for procaine and 0.3 $\mu mol.ml.h^{-1}$ for tetracaine. A correlation exists between the rate of metabolism of the various amino esters and their relative potential for producing systemic toxicity. Chloroprocaine, which undergoes the most rapid hydrolysis, is the least toxic of the ester type agents, while tetracaine, which shows the slowest rate of hydrolysis, is the most potentially toxic. Although these differences are due in part to the rate of hydrolysis, they may also be related to the difference in the inherent anaesthetic potency between tetracaine and chloroprocaine. Because the major portion of an injected dose of an amino ester undergoes hydrolysis in plasma, little is found in the urine.

The amino amide agents are metabolised primarily in the liver and there is considerable variation in their rates of hepatic degradation. Prilocaine, which is a secondary amine, undergoes the most rapid hepatic metabolism. Studies in man have shown that initially 80% of lidocaine, etidocaine and bupivacaine were cleared in a single passage through the liver. However, the hepatic clearance of bupivacaine quickly fell to approximately 50%, whereas the clear-

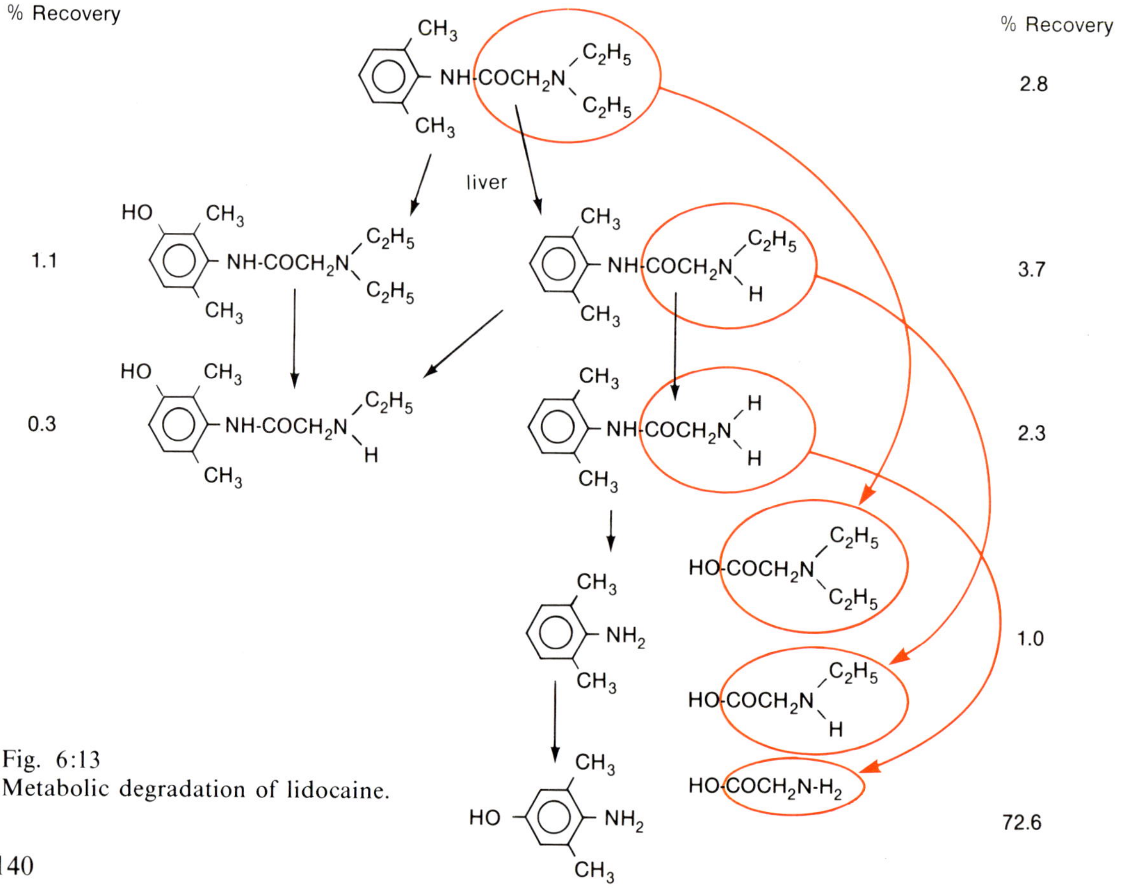

Fig. 6:13
Metabolic degradation of lidocaine.

ance of lidocaine and etidocaine remained at the 80% level. These studies suggest that bupivacaine is metabolised at a significantly lower rate than any of the other amino amides. Some degradation of the amide compounds may also take place in tissues other than the liver. The formation of certain metabolites has been observed following incubation of prilocaine with kidney slices. Again, the rapid disappearance of prilocaine from blood is probably due to its rapid rate of tissue redistribution related to its low plasma protein binding, its rapid metabolism by the liver and its ability to be metabolised by other organs such as the kidney. This favourable distribution/metabolic profile of prilocaine is responsible for its relatively low systemic toxicity.

The metabolism of the amide type agents is more complex than that of the ester drugs (Fig. 6:13). Although many of the metabolites of the various amino amides have been identified, the complete metabolic pathways for all compounds in this class have not been fully elucidated.

Fig. 6:14 Relationship between the plasma half life of lidocaine in young and old subjects.

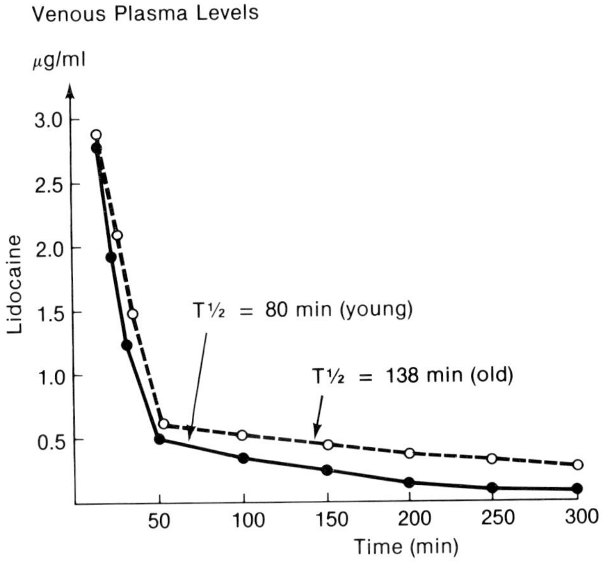

Most metabolic studies have been concerned with lidocaine. The main metabolic pathway for this agent in man involves de-ethylation to monoethylglycinexylidide (MEGX), which is subsequently hydrolysed to xylidine. The amino amides are almost completely metabolised prior to excretion, less than 5% of the parent drug being found in the urine. The major portion of the injected agent appears in the urine in the form of various metabolites.

Pharmacokinetic alterations

The uptake, distribution and elimination of local anaesthetic agents may be altered by a variety of clinical factors, including age, cardiac function, hepatic function, renal function and drug interaction.

Patient age can significantly influence the physiological disposition of local anaesthetic agents. Human volunteers, 22-26 years of age, had a mean half-life of lidocaine of 80.6 min, compared with a half-life of 138.6 min in subjects 61-71 years of age (Fig. 6:14). Pharmacokinetic studies of various amide local anaesthetics have revealed that the half-life of most of the amino amides is significantly prolonged in newborns (Table 6:3). Studies in newborn lambs with lidocaine and etidocaine suggest that the prolonged half-life is not due to a decrease in hepatic metabolism as a result of immature enzyme systems, but rather to an increased volume of distribution. However, mepivacaine, which has a half-life in adults of approximately 90 min, is reported to possess a half-life of 9 h in newborns, which may indeed represent an inability of the foetal liver to metabolise this agent.

The rate of lidocaine disappearance from blood is markedly prolonged in patients with decreased cardiac output, e.g., those with congestive heart failure (Fig. 6:15). The prolonged half-life of lidocaine in such patients is probably due to decreased hepatic blood flow, resulting in a decrease in hepatic uptake and metabolism.

Table 6:3
Comparative Biological Half-Lives of Amide Local Anaesthetics in Adults and Neonates

	T ½ (hours)	
Agent	Adult	Neonate
Lidocaine	1.5-1.8	3-3.5
Mepivacaine	1.5-3.0	8.6-9.0
Etidocaine	2.6	6.4
Bupivacaine	3.5	8.1

The rate of degradation of the amino amide local anaesthetics will be markedly influenced by the hepatic function of the individual patient. Significantly higher blood levels of the amino amides occur in patients in whom liver blood flow is abnormally low, or in whom liver function is poor or non-existent. An average half-life of lidocaine of 1.4 h was found in normal volunteers, compared with 7.3 h in patients with hepatitis (Fig. 6:16). Following recovery of liver function in these patients, the half-life of lidocaine returned to normal values. Although the amino esters are hydrolysed in plasma by pseudocholinesterase, this enzyme requires normal hepatic function for its production. Patients with advanced liver

Fig. 6:15 Relationship between the plasma half life of lidocaine in patients with normal cardiac function and patients in cardiac failure.

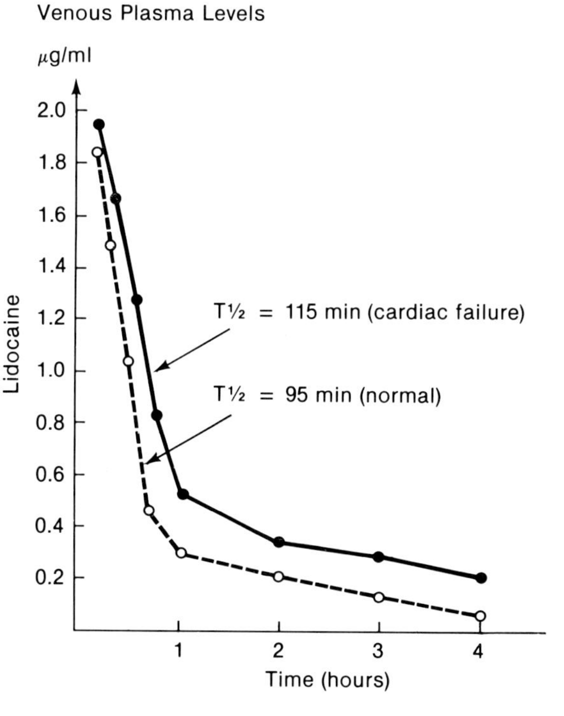

disease have shown a significant decrease in the rate of hydrolysis of procaine. Thus, patients with hepatic impairment will eliminate all local anaesthetic agents at a slower rate, which will tend to increase the potential systemic toxicity of these agents if repeated doses are given.

Although both the amino esters and amino amides are either hydrolysed in plasma or metabolised in liver prior to renal excretion, renal function is important in the removal of the degradation products. The half-life of lidocaine and its primary metabolite, monoethylglycinexylidide, is unaffected by the presence of renal failure. However, the disappearance rate of the secondary metabolite of lidocaine, glucine xylidide, is markedly delayed in patients with renal failure (Fig. 6:17).

Fig. 6:16 Relationship between the plasma half life of lidocaine in patients with acute hepatitis and following recovery from hepatitis.

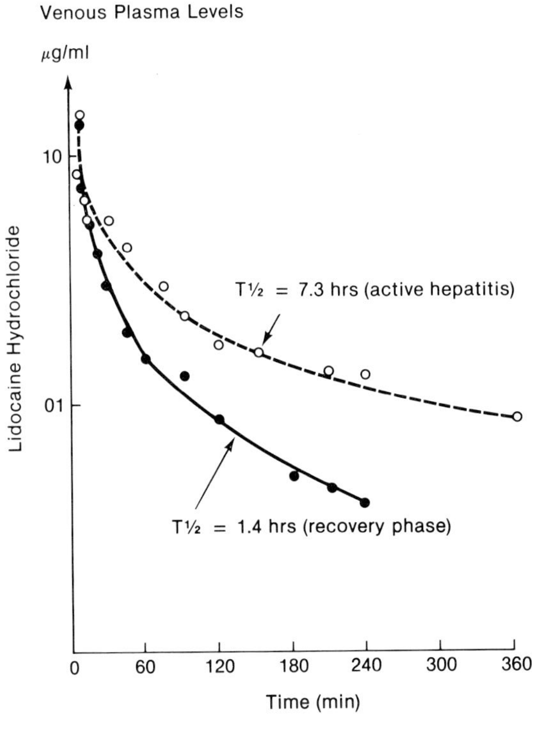

Fig. 6:17 Venous plasma levels of lidocaine, monoethylglycine xylidide (MEGX), and glycine xylidide (GX) in a patient with acute renal failure.

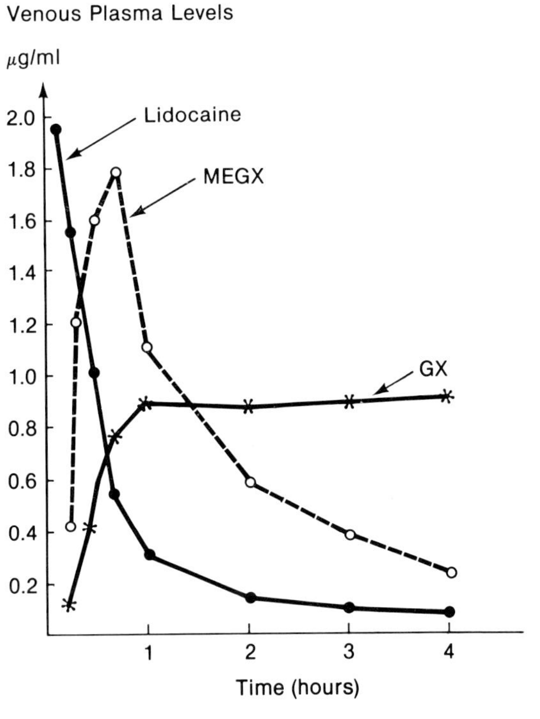

A number of interactions between local anaesthetic agents and other drugs exist. These interactions primarily alter the pharmacokinetic properties of local anaesthetics and thereby influence their potential systemic toxicity. Any agent which alters hepatic blood flow will affect the uptake and clearance of local anaesthetics by the liver. For example, isoproterenol, which increases hepatic blood flow, decreases the half-life of lidocaine, while norepinephrine, which decreases hepatic blood flow, prolongs it (Fig. 6:18). Cimetidine also reduces liver blood flow and prolongs the elimination half-life of lidocaine. Propranolol, which apparently is metabolised by the same hepatic enzyme system involved in the degradation of the amino amides, significantly prolongs the hepatic clearance of lidocaine (Fig. 6:19). Conversely, agents which cause hepatic enzyme induction, such as barbiturates, will increase the rate of metabolism of lidocaine (Fig. 6:19).

Changes in plasma cholinesterase levels or activity will alter the rate of hydrolysis of amino ester agents. Competition does exist between amino ester agents and neuromuscular blocking agents which depend on pseudocholinesterase for their hydrolysis. Prolonged apnoea has been observed when amino esters and depolarising types of neuromuscular blocking agents

Fig. 6:18 Relationship between the rate of disappearance of lidocaine from plasma in the presence of infusions of norepinephrine or isoproterenol.

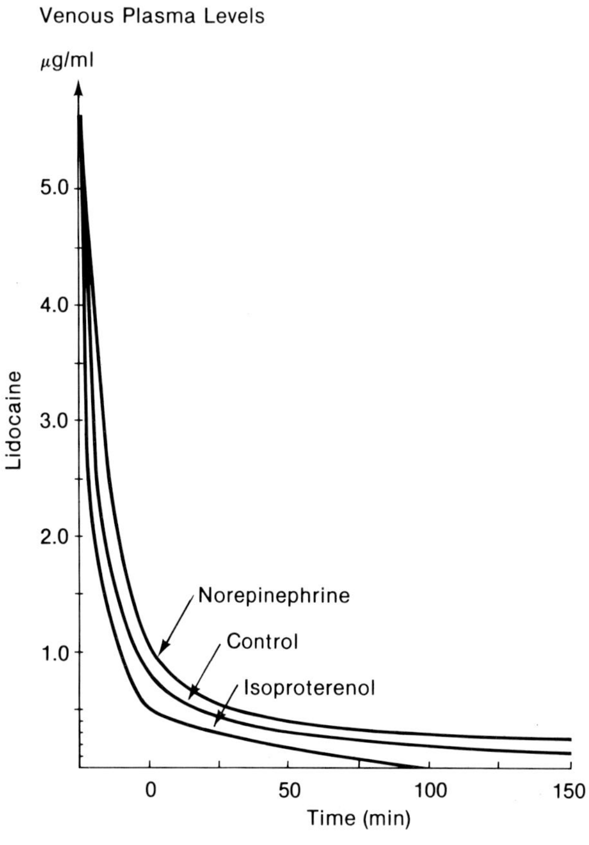

Fig. 6:19 Rate of disappearance of lidocaine from plasma in the presence of propranolol and barbiturate.

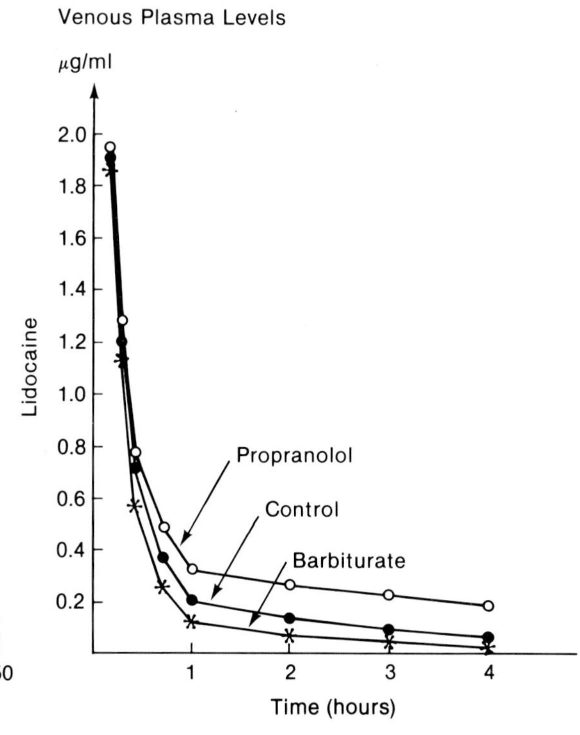

were administered concomitantly to animals. The duration of action of the amino esters has been shown to be prolonged in patients with atypical pseudocholinesterase.

In summary, the uptake, distribution and elimination of local anaesthetic agents are particularly important in terms of determining their potential systemic toxicity. Absorption is a function of the site of injection, the total dosage administered, the inclusion of a vasoconstrictor agent with the local anaesthetic and the specific local anaesthetic agent employed. The local anaesthetic agents are distributed throughout total body water. However, the rate of tissue redistribution appears to be primarily a function of the degree of plasma protein binding of the various local anaesthetics. The metabolism of local anaesthetic agents varies as a function of their chemical structure. The amino esters are hydrolysed in plasma by pseudocholinesterase, whereas the amino amides are degradated in the liver by microsomal enzymes. Differences in the rate of degradation of the various agents will influence their potential systemic toxicity. Chloroprocaine is the least toxic of all the local anaesthetics owing to its rapid rate of hydrolysis in plasma by cholinesterase. Prilocaine is the least toxic of the amino amides, mainly because of its rapid rate of both tissue redistribution and hepatic metabolism.

Systemic toxicity of local anaesthetic agents

Although the primary pharmacological action of local anaesthetic agents is the inhibition of the excitation conduction process in peripheral nerves, all excitable membranes, such as exist in heart, brain and neuromuscular junction, will be affected by local anaesthetic agents if they achieve a sufficient tissue concentration. Epidural anaesthesia if properly performed, does not usually result in blood levels of local anaesthetics sufficient to cause systemic effects. However, accidental intravascular injection or the administration of an excessive amount of local anaesthetic into the epidural space can result in blood and tissue levels which will cause profound systemic effects.

Effects on the central nervous system

The central nervous system is particularly susceptible to the systemic actions of local anaesthetic agents. The signs and symptoms of CNS toxicity are as follows. Initially feelings of numbness of the lips and tongue, light-headedness and dizziness are usually reported, followed frequently by visual and auditory disturbances such as difficulty in focusing and tinnitus. Other subjective CNS symptoms include disorientation and occasional feelings of drowsiness. Objective signs of an excitatory CNS effect include shivering, muscular twitching and tremors, involving at first muscles of the face and distal parts of the extremities. This may progress to generalised convulsions of a tonic-clonic nature. If a sufficiently large dose of a local anaesthetic agent is administered systemically, these initial signs of CNS excitation are rapidly followed by a state of generalised CNS depression. Seizure activity ceases and respiratory depression ensues. Ultimately respiratory arrest occurs.

Attempts to utilise the electroencephalogram to monitor CNS activity following administration of local anaesthetic agents have not proven to be of clinical value. In some subjects, the appearance of slow waves on the EEG, an increased amount of delta theta activity and decreased alpha activity have been correlated with early signs of CNS stimulation. In general, however, there does not appear to be a good correlation between changes in EEG activity and subjective symptoms of CNS excitation. EEG studies in animals indicate that the amygdala is most sensitive to the action of local anaesthetic agents. The mechanism for the excitatory effect of local anaesthetics in the brain is believed to involve the selective blockade of inhibitory pathways in the cerebral cortex, which allows facilitory neurons to function in an unopposed fashion, resulting in an increase in excitatory activity which leads to convulsions. Larger doses of local anaesthetics would tend to inhibit both inhibitory and facilitory pathways, resulting in a generalised state of CNS depression.

The potential CNS toxicity of local anaesthetic drugs is related to their potency (Table 6:4). For example, in dogs a dose of approximately 20 $mg.kg^{-1}$ of lidocaine was required to produce convulsions, compared with doses of 8 $mg.kg^{-1}$ of etidocaine and 5 $mg.kg^{-1}$ of bupivacaine. Thus, the relative CNS toxicity of bupivacaine, etidocaine and lidocaine is approximately 4:2:1, which is similar to the relative potency of these agents for the production of epidural anaesthesia in man. Studies in monkeys have shown that bupivacaine produces convulsions at a plasma level of approximately 4.5 $\mu g.ml^{-1}$, whereas lidocaine-induced convulsions were observed at a mean blood level of 25 $\mu g.ml^{-1}$. Studies in man in which blood levels of local anaesthetics have been determined at the time of either subjective symptoms of CNS excitation in volunteers or frank convulsions occurring during accidental intravenous injection, have also shown that a correlation exists between the local anaesthetic activity of these agents and their effect on the CNS. The speed of injection is also important. Blood levels that

Table 6:4

Relative in vivo Local Anaesthetic Potency and Intravenous Convulsant Dose (CD_{100}) of Various Agents in Animals

Agents	Relative Anesthetic Potency	Cat[1]	Dog[2]	Monkey[3]	Rabbit[4]
Procaine	1	35	-	-	15
Chloroprocaine	1	-	-	-	-
Mepivacaine	2	18	-	18	-
Prilocaine	2.	22	-	18	-
Lidocaine	2	15	22	14-22	6
Etidocaine	6	-	8	5	-
Bupivacaine	8	5	5	4	-
Tetracaine	8	-	4	-	3

1 Englesson (1973) 3 Munson et al (1970, 1975)
2 Liu et al (1982) 4 Sorel, Lejeune (1955)

Table 6:5

Effect of $PaCO_2$ on the Convulsive Threshold (CD_{100}) of Various Local Anaesthetics in Cats

	CD_{100} (mg/kg)		
Agent	$PaCO_2$ 25-40 torr	$PaCO_2$ 65-81 torr	% Change in CD_{100}
Procaine	35	17	- 51
Mepivacaine	18	10	- 44
Prilocaine	22	12	- 45
Lidocaine	15	7	- 53
Bupivacaine	5	2.5	- 50

Data derived from Englesson, 1973

increase rapidly cause toxic effects at lower concentrations than those which increase more slowly.

The acid base status of animals and patients can markedly affect the CNS activity of local anaesthetic agents (Table 6:5). In cats, the convulsive threshold of various local anaesthetics was decreased by approximately 50% when the $PaCO_2$ was elevated from 25-40 torr to 65-81 torr. The relationship between $PaCO_2$ and the effect of local anaesthetics on the CNS may be due to several factors. An elevation of $PaCO_2$ will enhance cerebral blood flow so that more anaesthetic agent is delivered to the brain. In addition, diffusion of CO_2 across the nerve membrane may result in a fall in intracellular pH, which will favour ionic trapping of local anaesthetics within neural cells.

Effects on the cardiovascular system

In general, the cardiovascular system appears to be more resistant to the effects of local anaesthetic agents than the central nervous system (Table 6:6). Studies in dogs and sheep have indicated that doses which cause significant cardiovascular depression are approximately three times higher than those which produce convulsions. For example, in sheep, there was a seven-fold difference between the blood levels of lidocaine required for irreversible cardiovascular collapse and the levels associated with convulsive activity. In dogs the ratio of cardiovascular toxicity to CNS activity varied from 3.5 to 6.7 for lidocaine, etidocaine, tetracaine, and bupivacaine. Although these studies indicate a greater resistance of the cardiovascular system as compared with the central nervous system, they also show that local anaesthetic agents can cause profound cardiovascular toxicity.

Table 6:6
Intravenous Dose of Local Anaesthetic Agents Required for Convulsive Activity (CD_{100}) and Irreversible Cardiovascular Collapse (LD_{100}) in Dogs

Agent	CD_{100}	LD_{100}	LD_{100}/CD_{100}
	mg.k^{-1}		Ratio
Lidocaine	22	76	3.5
Etidocaine	8	40	5.0
Bupivacaine	4	20	5.0
Tetracaine	5	27	5.4

Data derived from Liu et al (1982)

Cardiac effects

Electrophysiological studies in intact dogs and man indicate that as the dose and blood levels of lidocaine are increased, a prolongation of conduction time throughout various parts of the heart occurs. These are reflected in the electrocardiogram as an increase in the PR interval and QRS duration. Extremely high concentrations of local anaesthetics will depress spontaneous pacemaker activity in the sinus node resulting in sinus bradycardia and sinus arrest. A similar depression at the AV node also occurs, resulting in prolonged PR intervals and partial or complete AV dissociation.

Local anaesthetic agents also exert profound effects on the mechanical activity of cardiac muscle. In isolated cardiac tissue all local anaesthetics exert a dose dependent negative inotropic action which correlates with their local anaesthetic activity (Table 6:7).

The blood levels of local anaesthetics which obtain following epidural injection are rarely associated with signs of myocardial depression and/or a decrease in cardiac output. However, either an accidental rapid administration intravenously or an excessive dose can decrease myocardial contractility. For example, in dogs, bupivacaine and etidocaine caused a marked decrease in cardiac output at doses of approximately 5-10 mg.kg^{-1}, while with the less potent local anaesthetics mepivacaine, prilocaine and lidocaine, doses of 10-30 mg.kg^{-1} were required to produce the same effect.

Table 6:7

Comparison of Relative Anaesthetic Potency and Myocardial Depressant Effect of Local Anaesthetics

Agent	Relative Anaesthetic Potency	Concentration (μg.ml^{-1}) Required for 50% Depression of Atrial Contractility
Procaine	1	277
Chloroprocaine	2	102
Cocaine	4	56
Lidocaine	4	67
Prilocaine	4	42
Mepivacaine	4	55
Bupivacaine	16	6
Tetracaine	16	6

Data derived from Feldman et al. 1982.

Peripheral vascular effects

Local anaesthetic agents have a biphasic action on the smooth muscle of peripheral blood vessels. In vivo studies have demonstrated an initial stimulatory effect of local anaesthetic agents on vascular smooth muscle. For example, the intra-arterial administration of mepivacaine in human volunteers resulted in a decrease in forearm blood flow without any change in arterial pressure, suggesting that mepivacaine caused vasoconstriction. Similar studies with lidocaine also showed an increased tone in capacitance vessels, with less consistent effects on resistance vessels.

As the dose of local anaesthetic agent administered is increased, the stimulatory or vasoconstrictor action of these agents changes to one of inhibition and vasodilation. A comparison of the peripheral vascular effects of local anaesthetic agents has failed to demonstrate a good correlation between their relative anaesthetic potency and their ability to cause peripheral vasodilation. However, a correlation does appear to exist between the duration of action of these agents as local anaesthetics and their duration of vasodilation. The doses of local anaesthetics usually employed for epidural blockade produce a generalised state of vasodilation if accidentally administered intravenously.

In summary, the sequence of cardiovascular events that usually occurs following the accidental systemic administration of local anaesthetic agents is as follows: at relatively non-toxic blood levels of these agents, either no change in blood pressure or a slight increase in blood pressure may be observed. The slight increase in blood pressure may be related to an increase in cardiac output and heart rate which has been seen in some animal preparations and is believed to be due to an enhancement of sympathetic activity by these agents. In addition, the direct vasoconstrictor action of local anaesthetics on certain peripheral vascular beds at low concentrations may be responsible in part for a slight increase in systemic blood pressure. As the blood level of local anaesthetic agents approaches toxic concentrations, a fall in blood pressure is usually the first sign of a systemic effect. The hypotension appears to be correlated to the negative inotropic action of these agents, which results in a decrease in cardiac output and stroke volume. The initial reduction in blood pressure is transient and spontaneously reversible in most patients. However, if the amount of local anaesthetic administered is excessive, a profound and irreversible state of cardiovascular depression occurs. This is due not only to the negative inotropic action of the local anaesthetics, but also to massive peripheral vasodilation caused by a direct relaxant effect on vascular smooth muscle. At high concentrations the depressant effect of these agents on the excitability of cardiac tissue will also become evident as a decrease in sinus rate and AV conduction block. Ultimately, the combined peripheral vasodilation, decreased myocardial contractility and depressant effect on rate and conductivity will lead to cardiac arrest.

A general relationship exists between the potency of various agents as local anaesthetic drugs, and their depressant effect on the cardiovascular system. However, there is some evidence that the more potent, highly lipid-soluble and highly protein-bound local anaesthetic agents may be relatively more cardiotoxic than the less potent, less lipid-soluble and less protein-bound local anaesthetics. Several cases have been reported in which bupivacaine and etidocaine were associated with rapid and profound cardiovascular depression following accidental intravascular injection. In some cases severe cardiac arrhythmias were observed, and the cardiac depression appeared resistant to various therapeutic measures. Most of the reports of sudden cardiovascular collapse and death involved the use of 0.75% bupivacaine in obstetrical patients. As a result, the use of 0.75% bupivacaine for epidural anaesthesia in obstetrics is no longer recommended in several countries. The aetiology of these cardiac reactions is still not known.

A number of animal studies have been conducted to compare the cardiovascular effects of lidocaine and bupivacaine (Table 6:8). Cardiovascular depression produced by local anaesthetic agents in anaesthetised dogs appears to be related to the potency of the various drugs. On the other hand, as compared to lidocaine a narrow margin exists in mice between the dose of bupivacaine that will cause CNS toxicity and the dose that will cause cardiovascular toxicity. In sheep less difference exists between the dose of etidocaine and bupivacaine required for production of CNS and cardiovascular toxicity as compared with an agent such as lidocaine. In addition, it has been reported that bupivacaine can induce cardiac arrhythmias in unanaesthetised cats, dogs and sheep, whereas no such changes were observed with lidocaine (Fig. 6:20). Although the animal studies indicate that rapid intravenous injections of bupivacaine may cause ventricular arrhythmias, it is not clear whether this phenomenon is limited to bupivacaine or may occur with other local anaesthetics. The failure to observe arrhythmias with lidocaine may simply reflect the potent anti-arrhythmic properties of this agent. In view of the potential cardiotoxicity of bupivacaine and other agents, it has been recommended that every effort be made to avoid an accidental intravascular injection during the performance of an epidural block. The use of a test dose of a local anaesthetic with epinephrine is strongly recommended. In addition, slow injections or use of fractional dose techniques should be considered when performing epidural blocks.

The obstetrical patient may be more sensitive to the cardiodepressant action of local anaesthetics. As indicated above, most of the severe cardiac reactions to bupivacaine have occurred in obstetrical patients. In addition, it has been shown that the dose of bupivacaine required to produce cardiovascular collapse is lower in pregnant sheep than in non-pregnant sheep.

Changes in acid-base status will alter the potential cardiovascular toxicity of local anaesthetic agents. As mentioned previously, hypercarbia and acidosis will decrease the threshold of local anaesthetic agents for convulsive activity. Similarly, hy-

Table 6:8
Comparative Cardiotoxicity of Lidocaine and Bupivacaine

Species	Agent	Dose $mg.kg^{-1}$	Cardiac Event
Mouse	Lidocaine	133	Arrest
	Bupivacaine	58	Arrest
Cat	Lidocaine	4 $mg.kg.^{-1}min^{-1}$	-
	Bupivacaine	1 $mg.kg.^{-1}min^{-1}$	Ventricular Arrhythmias
Anesthetized dog	Lidocaine	76	Circulatory Collapse
	Bupivacaine	20	Circulatory Collapse
Awake dog	Lidocaine	11-16.5	---0/7
	Bupivacaine	3.4-5.1	V.F-2/7
Sheep	Lidocaine	5.7	-
	Bupivacaine	2.1	Ventricular Arrhythmias

percapnia, acidosis and hypoxia will tend to increase the cardiodepressant effect of local anaesthetic agents. It has been observed in some patients that marked hypercapnia, acidosis and hypoxia can occur very rapidly following seizure activity. Thus, the cardiovascular depression observed with the more potent agents such as bupivacaine may be related in part to the severe hypoxia and acid-base changes that occur following the administration of toxic doses of these agents.

Fig. 6:20 Electrocardiogram and arterial blood pressure in a dog following rapid intravenous administration of bupivacaine. (A) Indicates time of injection. (B) Indicates start of seizure activity which obscures the EKG and blood pressure recording for about 30 sec. (C) Indicates start of ventricular tachycardia leading to ventricular fibrillation.

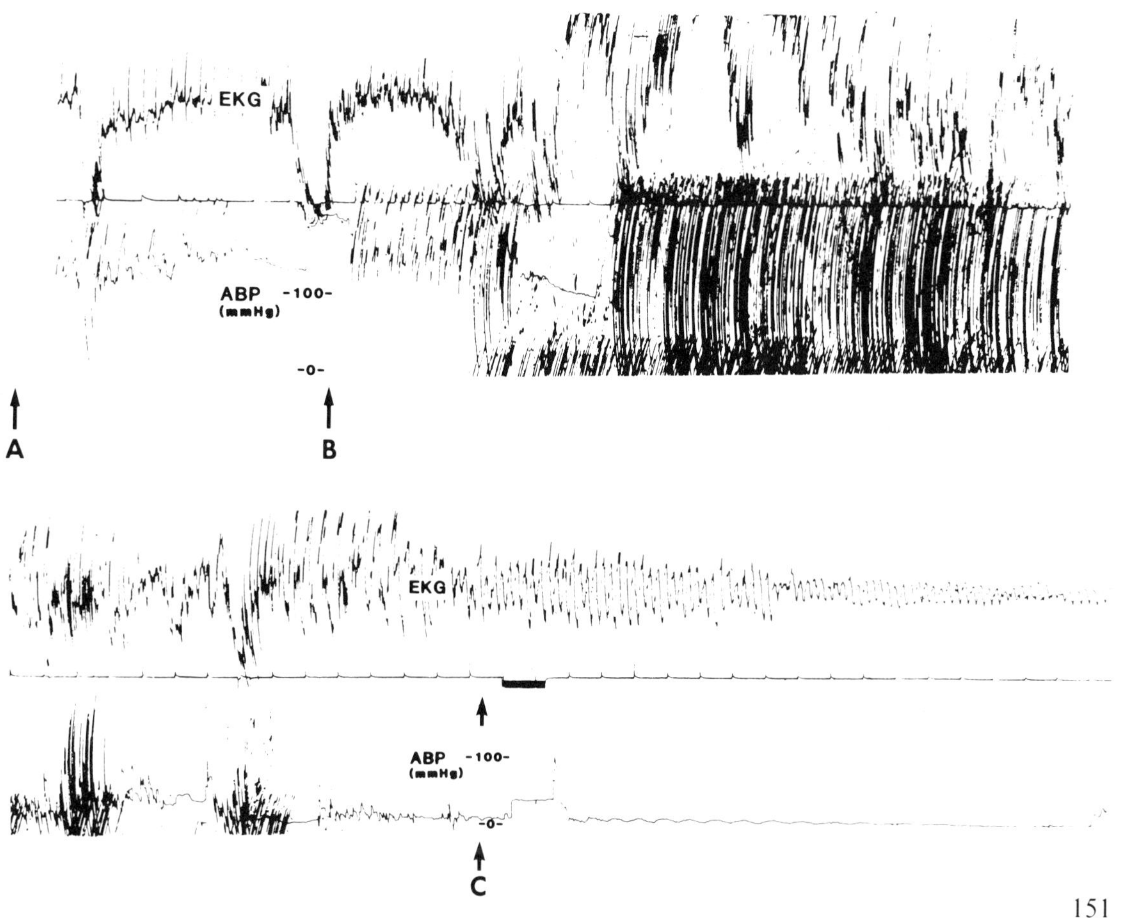

Other toxicological effects

Reports of allergic reactions, hypersensitivity or anaphylactic responses to local anaesthetic agents appear periodically. Unfortunately, systemic toxic reactions to local anaesthetic agents and vasovagal fainting are frequently misdiagnosed as representing allergic or hypersensitivity type reactions. The amino ester agents such as procaine have been shown to produce allergic type reactions. Since these agents are derivatives of paraaminobenzoic acid, which is known to be allergenic in nature, it is not surprising that a certain percentage of the population will demonstrate allergic reactions to this class of local anaesthetics. The advent of the amino amide local anaesthetics, which are not derivatives of paraaminobenzoic acid, markedly reduced the incidence of allergy to local anaesthetic drugs. Allergic reactions to the amino amides are extremely rare, although several cases have been reported in the literature in recent years which suggest that this class of agents can on rare occasions produce an allergic type phenomenon.

A technique of intradermal injection has been employed to study the frequency of allergy to both amino ester and amino amide local anaesthetics in patients with and without a presumptive history of local anaesthetic allergy. Positive skin reactions were observed in 25 of 60 patients with no previous allergic symptomatology. In all cases the cutaneous reactions occurred following the injection of an amino ester such as procaine, tetracaine and chloroprocaine. No cutaneous reactions occurred following the use of the amino amide agents, namely lidocaine, mepivacaine and prilocaine. Of 11 patients who had a history of alleged local anaesthetic allergy, eight showed a positive skin reaction to procaine, tetracaine or chloroprocaine. However, no positive cutaneous response was seen following lidocaine, mepivacaine or prilocaine. No signs of systemic anaphylaxis occurred in any of the subjects. It should be remembered that although the amino amide agents appear to be relatively free from allergic reactions, solutions of these drugs may contain a preservative, methylparaben, whose chemical structure is similar to that of paraaminobenzoic acid. It has been shown that patients in whom methylparaben was administered intradermally demonstrated a positive skin reaction.

One of the more unique systemic toxic effects of local anaesthetics involves the development of methaemoglobinaemia following the administration of relatively large doses of prilocaine. A correlation exists between the dose of prilocaine administered epidurally and the amount of methaemoglobin formation. Cyanosis may be observed following the epidural administration of 600 mg prilocaine or greater. Methaemoglobinaemia is believed to be due to the degradation of prilocaine to otoluidine, which in turn has the ability to enhance the oxidation of haemoglobin to methaemoglobin. Patients become cyanosed when 1 to 1.5 g% of methaemoglobin is formed in the blood, i.e., before there is a significant reduction in oxygen carrying capacity. Methaemoglobinaemia is spontaneously reversible, with regression occurring usually within 2-3 h. Alternatively, it can be reversed by the administration of methylene blue, 0.5-1 $mg.kg^{-1}$. While the formation of methaemoglobinaemia in healthy patients is of little clinical relevance, the use of prilocaine may be contraindicated in patients with severe anaemia or cardiac failure.

Treatment of systemic toxicity

Adverse reactions are usually due to an accidental intravascular injection of a local anaesthetic agent. The severity and duration of the toxic reaction depends on the amount of drug administered and the specific agent employed. Convulsions, which represent the most common serious adverse reaction, are usually transient in nature. In dogs, the duration of convulsive activity varied from 2.9 min in etidocaine-treated animals to 5.2 min when tetracaine was administered. The duration of toxic reactions is probably related to the pharmacokinetic properties of the different drugs. Local anaesthetics which possess relatively short pharmacokinetic half-lives, such as prilocaine, lidocaine, chloroprocaine and etidocaine, will produce toxic reactions of shorter duration compared with agents such as bupivacaine, which has a relatively long half-life.

The primary treatment of CNS toxicity should be directed towards maintaining adequate ventilation. During convulsions oxygen is being used at a high rate, and as respiration is usually inadequate, hypoxia and acidosis quickly develop. Therefore, every effort should be made to establish and maintain a patent airway, and to assist or control ventilation with oxygen. Frequently, no additional therapy is required since the convulsions are self-limiting. If they persist, the use of a central nervous system depressant drug is indicated. Thiopental (1-2 $mg.kg^{-1}$) is the most commonly employed agent to terminate persistent signs of CNS excitation. It is highly effective and has the advantage of being easily available and familiar to all anaesthetists. Diazepam (0.1 - 0.2 $mg.kg^{-1}$) has been recommended but it is much slower in its effect than thiopental and this makes the estimation of dosage problematic. Moreover its duration of action is much more prolonged than is the case with thiopental. A rapidly acting, short-duration neuromuscular blocking agent such as succinylcholine may also be employed to abort a state of generalised convulsions. In such a situation, the patient should be intubated in order to control respiration adequately.

Signs of cardiovascular depression require immediate therapy. Hypotension may respond to intravenous fluids, but persistent hypotension requires the use of vasopressor agents. Severe circulatory depression should be treated with agents which exert a positive inotropic action as well as a peripheral vasoconstrictor effect, e.g., ephedrine (0.2 - 0.4 $mg.kg^{-1}$). If cardiac arrest occurs, immediate institution of cardiopulmonary resuscitation is imperative. If ventricular fibrillation occurs, high levels of electrical energy may be necessary to restore sinus rhythm.

In those rare situations in which signs of dermal allergic reactions occur, administration of an intravenous antihistamine such as diphenhydramine (50 mg) may prove useful. Immediate therapy should be instituted if signs of anaphylaxis occur. Hypotension again requires the administration of a vasopressor agent which possesses a positive inotropic and a peripheral vasoconstrictor action. Bronchoconstriction may be treated with adrenergic bronchodilators such as epinephrine or terbutaline or xanthine derivatives like aminophylline. Steroids such as hydrocortisone may also be of value in the treatment of anaphylactic reactions.

Toxic reactions can usually be prevented by the use of proper precautions regarding dosage of the local anaesthetic agent and avoidance of intravascular injections. However, resuscitation equipment should always be readily available during the performance of regional anaesthetic techniques in order to treat the occasional unavoidable adverse reaction that may occur.

Local tissue toxicity

The potential of epidurally administered local anaesthetic agents to cause localised nerve damage is very low. The spinal cord and spinal roots may be more vulnerable since they lack a connective tissue sheath. However, epidemiological studies on spinal anaesthesia indicate that localised neurotoxicity is not a major problem.

Some concern has been expressed regarding the potential neurotoxicity of chloroprocaine. The possibility that this agent can cause localised neural damage is based on the reports of prolonged neurological deficits in four patients following the epidural or accidental subarachnoid injection of large doses of this particular drug. Studies in animals have proven to be somewhat contradictory (Table 6:9). Chloroprocaine but not lidocaine was found to cause local toxic effects in an isolated rabbit vagus nerve preparation. However, rabbit sciatic nerves exposed to chloroprocaine for a period of 6 h did not reveal any histological signs of damage. Investigations were conducted in dogs in which chloroprocaine and bupivacaine were administered intra-

Table 6:9
Neurotoxicity of Local Anaesthetics
Animal Studies

Type of study	Investigator	Toxicity			
		Chloroproc.	Lido.	Bup.	Other solns.
Rabbit Vagus Nerve	Barsa	+ + +	0	-	-
Rabbit Sciatic Nerve	Pizzolato	0	0	-	-
Spinal Dog	Feldman	0	0	0	0
Spinal Dog	Ravindran	+ + +	-	0	0
Spinal Rabbit	Wang	+ + +	-	-	+ + +, 0
Spinal Sheep	Rosen	+	+	0	+
Spinal Monkey	Rosen	+	-	+	-

0 = no effect
+ = mild toxicity
+ + + = severe toxicity
- = not studied

thecally in doses sufficient to cause total spinal anaesthesia. Chloroprocaine produced permanent paralysis in approximately 30% of the animals, whereas none of the bupivacaine treated dogs showed evidence of such sequelae. Studies of a similar nature in sheep and monkeys have failed to show any difference in neurotoxicity between chloroprocaine and other local anaesthetics or control solutions. Paralysis which was observed in rabbits to which intrathecal chloroprocaine solutions were administered was believed to be related to sodium bisulphite, which is employed as an antioxidant in chloroprocaine solutions. Solutions of chloroprocaine without sodium bisulphite did not cause paralysis, whereas the sodium bisulphite alone was associated with paralysis. Studies in isolated nerves have shown that the combination of a low pH and bisulphite may be responsible for irreversible conduction blockade rather than the chloroprocaine itself (Table 6:10). However, it is obvious that epidural blockade should be performed with great care to avoid the accidental intrathecal injection of large amounts of local anaesthetics.

Table 6:10

Effect of Chloroprocaine (CP), pH and Bisulfite on Conduction in A and C Fibers of Rabbit Vagus Nerve

LA	pH	Bisulfite	Recovery Time (min)	
			A	C
3% Nesacaine	3.0	0.2%	∞	∞
3% CP	3.0	0.2%	∞	∞
3% CP	7.2	-	60	120
3% CP	3.2	-	60	120
3% CP	7.3	0.2%	60	120
3% Nesacaine	7.3	0.2%	60	60
N-Saline	7.0	0.2%	-	-
N-Saline	3.3	0.2%	∞	∞

— = no block
∞ = irreversible block
Nesacaine is commercially available CP.

Side effects of epidural opioids

The administration of opioids into the epidural space can effectively inhibit the conduction of nociceptive impulses within the spinal cord, but is not associated with any signs of motor weakness or hypotension due to sympathetic blockade. However, various side-effects have been reported following the epidural use of these agents: pruritus, nausea and vomiting, urinary retention and respiratory depression.

Pruritus

Intense itching has been reported in approximately 10%-30% of patients following the epidural administration of various narcotic analgesics. Although the analgesia appears to be segmental in nature, the phenomenon of pruritus does not appear to be limited to the dermatomal segments affected by the epidural opioids. The intense itching frequently occurs in the facial region and then spreads to other areas of the body. The mechanism responsible for the pruritic effect has not as yet been elucidated. Although some opioids such as morphine are capable of causing the release of histamine, it is not certain whether this is responsible for the observed pruritus, and the use of antihistaminics in reversing the pruritus following epidural opioids has not proved universally successful. However, it does appear that the parenteral administration of naloxone is capable of reversing this intense itching.

Nausea and vomiting

Nausea and vomiting have also been reported in approximately 10%-30% of patients receiving epidural opioids, usually within 1 h but sometimes as long as 6-10 h after injection. The early state of nausea and vomiting is probably related to the absorption of the narcotic analgesics from the epidural space which is similar to that observed following the intramuscular administration of these compounds. The delayed nausea and vomiting probably reflects the time required for diffusion of epidural opioids into the cerebrospinal fluid and the subsequent migration from the point of injection to the brain. It is believed that both the early and the delayed occurrence of nausea and vomiting is due to the stimulation of the vomiting centre in the area postrema, which lies in the floor of the fourth ventricle. Various anti-emetic agents have proven useful in the treatment of the nausea and vomiting. In addition, naloxone has also been effective.

Urinary retention

Urinary retention requiring catheterisation can persist for 10-20 h and appears to be more frequent in males. This side-effect has been observed in 10%-30% of patients receiving epidural opioids. The mechanism is not clear, but it is possible that the epidural opioids interfere with parasympathetic activity in the sacral area. Methacholine and parenteral naloxone have been reported to be useful in treating urinary retention.

Respiratory depression

The most serious side effect reported following the use of epidural narcotic analgesics is the production of respiratory depression, which may be life threathening in certain patients (Fig. 6:21). As with nausea and vomiting, respiratory depression may occur as an early phenomenon or be delayed. There is a progressive decrease in respiratory rate, leading ultimately to apnoea and in addition a decreased respiratory response to elevated $PaCO_2$ levels. The early period of respiratory depression occurs approximately 1 h following the epidural administration and is believed to be related to the vascular absorption and the subsequent migration of the agents across the blood-brain barrier to the respiratory centre in the region of the fourth ventricle. This early period of respiratory depression is not considered as serious as the late phase of respiratory depression since patients are usually carefully monitored for several

Fig. 6:21 $PaCO_2$ levels 12 hours following the epidural administration of varying doses of morphine.

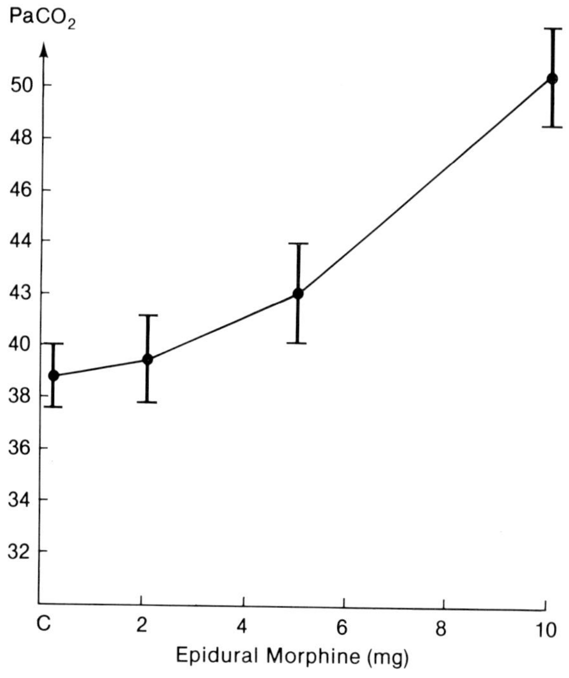

hours following the use of epidural opioids. Thus, any decrease in respiratory rate will usually be quickly recognised and the appropriate therapy instituted. The late phase of respiratory depression has been reported to occur some 6-12 h following the administration of these agents into the epidural space. This delay is probably related again to the migration of the opioids from the epidural space into the cerebrospinal fluid and subsequent diffusion to the fourth ventricle, where direct depression of the respiratory centre occurs.

Fortunately, respiratory depression appears to be less frequent than the other side-effects, such as pruritus, nausea and vomiting and urinary retention. It also seems to occur more frequently (about 1 in 200 administrations) in the treatment of acute postoperative pain. Respiratory depression has rarely been observed when epidural opioids have been employed for the treatment of chronic pain. It is believed that patients with chronic pain who have been exposed to parenteral opioids for a long period of time develop a tolerance to opioids administered epidurally. Late respiratory depression has been observed more commonly following the use of epidural morphine than with the other opioids. This may simply represent the fact that this agent has been the one employed most often. On the other hand, owing to its low lipid solubility, morphine may spread rostrally more readily than other opioids once it enters the subarachnoid space. The use of analgesics which are more lipophilic, such as fentanyl and pethidine, has only rarely been associated with respiratory depression. Since these agents move more freely between the epidural and subarachnoid space and since they also may be taken up to a great degree by the epidural fat, less drug may reach the respiratory centres in the brain. Respiratory depression is relatively uncommon following the use of epidural opioids alone. However, when combined with i.m or i.v. opioids, the incidence of respiratory depression increases markedly. Therefore great care should be taken in using systemic opioids in patients who have received epidural opioids within the previous 24 h.

Fortunately naloxone has proven to be effective in rapidly reversing the respiratory depression associated with epidural opioids, and it does not reverse the analgesic effects. It is not known whether the administration of naloxone into the epidural or intrathecal area will reverse the analgesic activity of the opioids.

In summary, the epidural use of opioid analgesics is an effective means of controlling both acute pain, such as occurs during the immediate postoperative period, and various forms of chronic pain. However, these agents are not without side-effects which are potentially lethal. Approximately 10%-30% of patients report pruritus, nausea and vomiting, and urinary retention. Severe respiratory depression, particularly that which occurs on a delayed basis, represents the most dangerous side-effect associated with the epidural use of these agents. Intravenous or intramuscular naloxone has proven to be highly successful in the treatment of all the side-effects associated with the use of epidural opiates, without reversing the analgesia.

Technique related complications

Cardiovascular complications

Hypotension

This is the commonest cardiovascular complication of epidural anaesthesia and results primarly from the widespread sympathetic blockade. The haemodynamic effects of epidural blockade are discussed on page 48. In general, sympathetic blockade will not cause an excessive fall in arterial pressure in normovolaemic patients not suffering from cardiovascular disease. Epidural blockade up to T_{10} seldom causes any decrease in arterial pressure and even with blocks into the upper thoracic segments, decreases greater than 10-20 mm Hg are uncommon in healthy patients. This is because, at rest, sympathetic tone is not high and the degree of vasodilation produced is only modest. If on the other hand there is a reduced cardiac output, e.g., due to hypovolaemia or inferior vena caval occlusion, such that high sympathetic tone is required to maintain arterial pressure, then the epidural block may well produce a severe degree of hypotension.

Hypotension is usually believed to be related to the inhibition of the sympathetic arterial vasoconstrictors and cardiac accelerator fibres. However, the capacitance vessels, i.e., the veins, are also under the influence of the sympathetic nervous system, blockade of which removes the ability of the veins to constrict. Capacitance will thus increase and the veins become dilatable. It is often thought that, because of this, the veins will fill with blood and the cardiac output will decrease. This however will only occur if there is a physical impediment to the flow of venous blood, such as gravity (the head up position) or inferior vena caval occlusion. Venomotor control, which is so important when the upright posture is adopted, is lost during sympathetic blockade, but cardiac output will be largely unaffected if the patient remains supine or slightly head down.

The circulation is also under the influence of the vagus nerves which exert their effect mainly through the cardiac branches, slowing the heart rate and opposing the action of the sympathetic nerves. In addition the vagi control the gastrointestinal musculature, increased activity in which demands an increase in blood supply and the diversion of part of the cardiac output. The vagi, being cranial nerves, are not affected by epidural blockade. Hence the increased gastrointestinal activity and bradycardia may potentiate the hypotension associated with sympathetic blockade.

Occasionally the vagus nerves become overactive, possibly as a result of the alteration in sympathetic/parasympathetic balance. A vasovagal attack then develops. This is characterised by marked bradycardia (even temporary cardiac arrest) and abnormal gastrointestinal activity such as nausea and vomiting. Hypotension may be rapid and profound and vasovagal attacks are responsible for most of the dramatic falls in blood pressure occasionally seen in epidural anaesthesia. During an attack there is complete cessation of sympathetic activity. The very low blood pressure is due to reductions both in cardiac output and peripheral resistance.

Light general anaesthesia, if added to an epidural block, can alter considerably the cardiovascular effects of the block. Hypotension occurs more frequently and is more profound, presumably because peripheral resistance is further decreased, either by inhibiting the vasoconstrictor effects of unblocked segments, or by direct vasodilatation of the arterioles. The hypotension is not usually accompanied by a commensurate fall in cardiac output unless the depth of the general anaesthesia is excessive. This accounts for the relative safety of hypotension deliberately induced by combining high blockade with general anaesthesia.

Although general anaesthesia increases the incidence and degree of hypotension, it has the great advantage of largely suppressing vagal overactivity and vasovagal attacks seldom, if ever, occur in unconscious patients. High blocks can cause bradycardia but this is not as sudden or profound as is seen with a vasovagal faint.

It should always be remembered that hypotension is a symptom and not a disease entity. It results from a decrease in peripheral resistance or cardiac output or both. If output is relatively unaffected no harm will result, unless in a conscious patient a vasovagal attack is precipitated. Although hypotension decreases coronary filling pressure, cardiac work is also reduced to a like degree as afterload is decreased. While this is valid for patients with normal coronary vessels, the position is more problematic if there is coronary artery disease. Until better means are available of judging coronary blood flow and detecting areas of ischaemia, profound hypotension should be avoided particularly in elderly patients.

Treatment

Treatment for hypotension during epidural anaesthesia will depend on proper assessment of the cause of the lowered arterial pressure. If the hypotension is sudden and accompanied by bradycardia and nausea, then vagal overactivity should be suspected. Atropine is often given in this situation but it is much less effective than a vasopressor (vide infra).

The low pressure is more usually due to a decreased peripheral resistance. This is the cause of hypotension due to sympathetic blockade or when a light general anaesthetic has been added. It is relatively benign and forms the basis of induced hypotension with high epidural or spinal blockade. As such it can be employed to reduce blood loss in operations where this is considered beneficial. The pulse rate will usually be in the normal range (60 - 80 beats/min) though young patients may develop a mild tachycardia (80 - 120 beats/min). If the block is high enough to affect the cardiac accelerator fibres, then a mild bradycardia 50 - 60 beats/min) may result. The degree of hypotension requiring active treatment is largely a matter of opinion. Rules of thumb such as a 30% fall in systolic pressure have little evidence for their validity. Moreover the treatment can raise the pressure at different rates, vasopressors being rapid and intravenous fluids being slow. Thus there is a degree of judgement required in all cases.

Vasopressor agents

These may be a pure α-adrenoreceptor stimulator, e.g., phenylephrine given as an i.v. infusion, or combined α- and β-stimulators, e.g., ephedrine 10-30 mg i.v. or i.m. Methoxamine, which is both an α-stimulator and a β-blocker, causes reversal of the hypotension and a bradycardia, with a reduction in cardiac output. The resultant balance between oxygen supply and demand of the myocardium has not been determined and the drug is less popular than it was. All these agents are very rapid in their effect and when given intravenously care should be taken to avoid hypertension. If given intramuscularly their action is slower and more prolonged. Thus combined i.v. and i.m. injection will raise the pressure quickly and maintain it for a longer time. Many authorities prefer to give them intramuscularly prophylactically at the time of epidural injection, but as only a minority of patients will become hypotensive this may be overcautious.

Posture

All patients whose arterial pressure falls should be tilted head down to avoid pooling of blood in the legs. A useful rise in pressure due to increased cardiac output usually follows this simple manoeuvre. If the hypotension is thought to be due to inferior vena caval occlusion, then this must be relieved by an appropriate change in posture.

Intravenous fluids

The use of fluids to increase circulating blood volume will counteract hypotension even in patients not clinically hypovolaemic. Crystalloids arc just as effective as colloids in the short term and can be eliminated quickly if renal function is adequate. If treatment of the hypotension is not urgent, the rapid infusion (250 - 500 ml of crystalloid in 15-30 min) will usually be effective. In patients with normal hydration, it is seldom necessary to give more than 1-1.5 l of fluid during the 1-3 h of the block.

It will be seen that only vasopressors are capable of reversing the prime cause of this type of hypotension, i.e., the decrease in peripheral resistance. Posture and fluids work by increasing cardiac output. The effect of fluids therefore is less pronounced and less rapid than vasopressors.

Cardiac arrest

This is a rare complication of epidural block but may result from severe hypotension and consequent myocardial ischaemia. The hypotension may be the result of a severe vasovagal attack or due to a high block in a severely hypovolaemic patient. In such cases the patient should respond to normal cardiopulmonary resuscitation with added vasopressor and fluids as appropriate.

More seriously, cardiac arrest may follow a degree of hypotension in a patient with coronary artery disease. The relationship between arterial pressure, coronary blood flow and myocardial work has been alluded to above. Many authorities would insist on reversing hypotension as and when it occurs. However, there may be advantages in leaving the arterial pressure on the low side, e.g., to reduce bleeding. In such cases the ECG should be carefully monitored using the V5 electrode position which can detect early abnormalities in the ST segment.

Finally cardiac arrest may occur as a result of a toxic reaction to the local anaesthetic (see p. 148). Immediate institution of cardiopulmonary resuscitation is imperative.

Respiratory complications

Epidural block seldom has any profound effect on quiet normal respiration. Several studies have failed to show any significant changes in blood gases even at high levels of blockade. Although high blocks may paralyse the intercostal muscles, the diaphragm is able, in the great majority of patients, to achieve adequate respiration. If for some reason the diaphragm cannot achieve this, e.g., in gross obesity, then respiration may have to be supported.

Very high blocks which would affect the nerve supply to the diaphragm (C_{3-5}) would, of course, render the patient apnoeic. They are usually due to accidental subarachnoid injection (vide infra) but occasionally occur with abnormally high spread in the epidural space.

Occasionally the patient may complain of inability to breathe during a vasovagal attack, and this can be misdiagnosed as an accidental subarachnoid block. It is probably due to the low cardiac output causing air hunger and quickly responds to measures which increase the output.

Total or high spinal blockade

This is the most feared complication of epidural block and is due to the inadvertent subarachnoid injection of an excessive amount of local anaesthetic. It does have very profound effects on the patient yet no permanent harm should ensue if proper management is instituted. Every anaesthetist undertaking epidural block should be able to recognise total or high spinal blockade and be prepared to treat it promptly.

The dose of local anaesthetic required for epidural block is much greater than that for spinal block, and it is easy to see how a very high spread of blockade may result from misplaced injections.

Clinical features

Spinal anaesthesia has a more rapid onset than epidural block and this is especially so if the dosage is excessive. Thus a profound degree of sensory and motor blockade developing within 1-5 min of injection, and to a very high dermatome level, will be the usual presenting signs. If the blockade reaches the upper cervical segments then respiratory arrest due to diaphragmatic paralysis will result. Unlike the epidural space, which stops at the foramen magnum, the spinal subarachnoid space communicates freely with the cerebral subarachnoid space, including the ventricular system of the brain. Should local anaesthetic reach the cranium then a total nerve paralysis will ensue. The patient will become unconscious, respiration will cease and severe hypotension will develop. Dilatation of the pupils will occur due to cranial nerve block.

High spinal blockade may be confused with:

High epidural blockade. This can occur but is much slower in onset.

Subdural injection. This can also cause a very high block but again is somewhat slower in onset.

Vasovagal attack. This can cause unconsciousness with dilated pupils and absent pulses. It is usually short-lived, however, and is preceded by a progressive sinus bradycardia.

Low cardiac output. If, as may occur with a vasovagal attack or with inferior vena caval occlusion or both, there is a marked decrease in cardiac output, then the patient may complain of feeling faint and having difficulty in breathing.

Prevention

Insertion into the subarachnoid space of the large bore needles which are usually used for epidural block is almost always recognised at the time by the rapid escape of cerebrospinal fluid (Fig. 6:22). Less rapid escape must be distinguished from that of the fluid used in detecting the epidural space. This can be done simply by allowing the fluid to drip onto the anaesthetist's skin (the back of the wrist is very suitable) and estimating the temperature. If cold, the fluid escaping is the injected solution; if warm, it is probably cerebrospinal fluid.

Where any doubt exists, a test dose of local anaesthetic may be given. If a small dose causes an obvious and widespread degree of nerve block in a few minutes then it must be presumed that the needle or catheter is in the subarachnoid space. However, a reasonable dose must be given and adequate time allowed for it to work. Thus 3-5 ml of 2% lidocaine or 0.5% bupivacaine allowed 5 min to produce an effect is required. It should be remembered that many case reports of accidental total spinal blocks have appeared in which inadequate test doses were given. Perhaps the ideal solution for a test dose is a hyperbaric spinal solution of local anaesthetic. One to two millilitres of such a solution will cause a rapid and widespread nerve blockade if injected into the subarachnoid space, but little or no blockade if injected into the epidural space (see p. 98).

Fig. 6:22 Dural tap. Note rapid and unmistakeable leakage of cerebrospinal fluid.

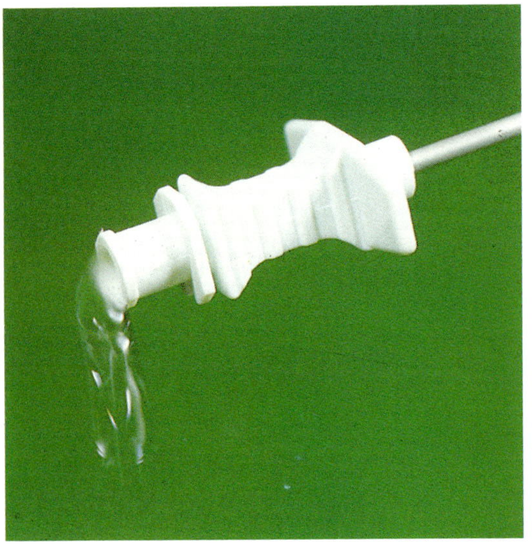

Treatment

This is simple in spite of the dramatic clinical picture of an apnoeic, unconscious and hypotensive patient. Oxygen must be given by artificial ventilation, aided, but not preceded by, endotracheal intubation. A vasopressor in dosage sufficient to normalise the blood pressure is also necessary, e.g., ephedrine 15-30 mg i.v. or phenylephrine by i.v. drip. The artificial respiration must be continued until spontaneous efforts resume. This may take a variable time depending on the drug and dose used. The decision whether or not to proceed with the planned surgery is a matter for individual judgement, but a total spinal block is not a contra-indication to surgery any more than is total paralysis due to a muscle relaxant.

Accidental subdural injection

The subdural space is only a potential space as the dura and arachnoid mater are separated only by a film of lymph. An injection of local anaesthetic into this space can therefore spread a considerable distance and will only be separated from the spinal nerves by the relatively thin arachnoid and pia mater. A block similar to a high or total spinal block may ensue, and the diagnosis can often only be made by a subsequent injection of radio-opaque dye. Fig. 6:23a and b shows a radiograph following the injection of 5 ml of radio-opaque dye. Note the very thin film of dye spreading cephalad for many segments.

Fig. 6:23 Radiographs a. Anteroposterior and b. Lateral, showing a subdural placement of dye. Note very high spread with confinement in the subdural space. (Kind permission of Dr. Alastair Lee).

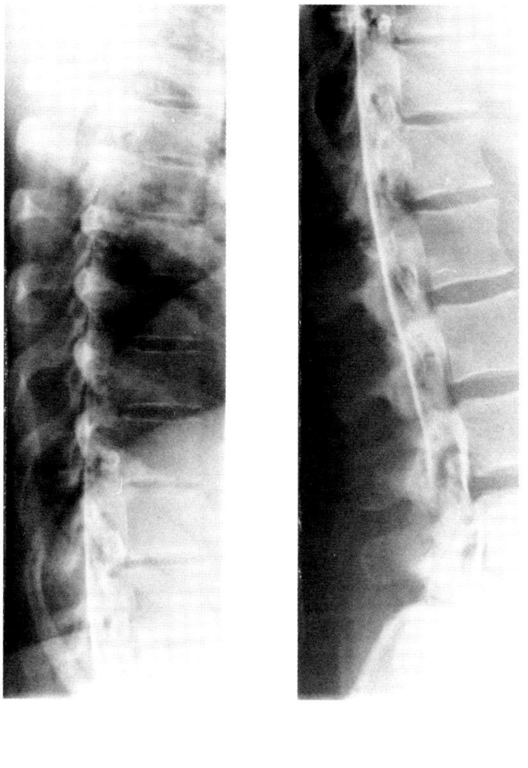

Reported cases seem to indicate that the onset of a subdural block takes rather longer than a subarachnoid injection, needing perhaps 20-30 min to become fully developed. The initial appearance of nerve block at some distance from the site of injection is also a clue as to the position of the needle or catheter. Thus a test dose may be followed by obvious anaesthesia in the upper thoracic or cervical area with no such anaesthesia in the lumbar area. The treatment of a fully developed subdural block is exactly the same as for a high spinal block.

Dural puncture

This is usually easy to diagnose as cerebrospinal fluid (CSF) escapes freely from the large bore needle (Fig. 6:22). The anaesthetist must then decide how he should proceed. If the proposed operation is of a duration which can be covered with a spinal anaesthetic, then a suitable dose of local anaesthetic should be injected to produce spinal anaesthesia.

If a nerve block of longer duration is required, the needle should be withdrawn and reinserted at an adjacent intervertebral space. Alternatively a catheter can be inserted into the subarachnoid space, and a continuous spinal block instituted. In any event, a spinal headache is likely to develop within the next 1-3 days.

Spinal headache

A typical spinal headache can follow puncture of the dura mater while attempting an epidural injection. The large size of needle generally used for epidural block ensures a high incidence of headache, of the order of 50%-75%. The prime cause of the headache is the leakage of CSF into the epidural space, causing a lowering of spinal CSF pressure, and the tendency of the brain to descend in the vertical position.

The headache is quite different from other headaches and presents few problems in diagnosis. It is very severe and related to posture, being worst in the upright and less in the supine position. It may be accompanied by signs of meningism, with a stiff painful neck. It is often accompanied by a marked degree of mental depression not seen with other types of headache. Spinal headache can appear any time up to 5 days after the dural puncture, depending on the time ambulation was resumed after the dural tap. The diagnosis may be missed when the delay is marked and sometimes the headache may not appear until after the patient has been discharged.

It should be differentiated from other causes of headache such as migraine or meningitis, though the history and clinical picture will seldom cause any great doubt.

Treatment may be conservative or active. The former consists of analgesics, maintaining the horizontal position and fluid loading. If the epidural catheter is still in place, a continuous infusion of saline can be made to raise the epidural pressure and prevent escape of CSF. It is tempting to start and persevere with conservative treatment on the basis that the condition is self-limiting and will eventually disappear. However, active treatment is so effective and free from complication that it is difficult to justify its delay for more than 24 h. Active treatment consists of injecting homologous blood into the epidural space, where it clots and presumably seals the dural puncture hole, i.e., it forms a "blood patch". It is done quite simply by inserting an epidural needle into the same or the adjacent intervertebral space to that used when dural puncture occurred and injecting 10-15 ml of the patient's own blood (Fig. 6:24). This should be withdrawn using full aseptic and antiseptic precautions and injected without delay into the epidural space. No anticoagulant should, of course, be added to the blood.

The results of "blood patching" are highly gratifying. The headache disappears rapidly (often almost immediately after the injection) and the patient can resume normal activity. This rapid relief is possibly due to the injected blood reducing the volume of the epidural space and increasing cerebrospinal fluid pressure. Unlike saline, it will only be absorbed very slowly. It is wise to keep the patient supine for an hour or so to ensure the blood remains at the puncture site until after it has clotted.

Occasionally the injection of blood has to be repeated. It is clearly advisable that the person carrying out the treatment is experienced and will not create a second dural puncture.

Animal experiments and the results of many years experience worldwide have attested to the relative safety of blood patching.

Fig. 6:24 Injection of homologous blood into the epidural space: The "blood patch".

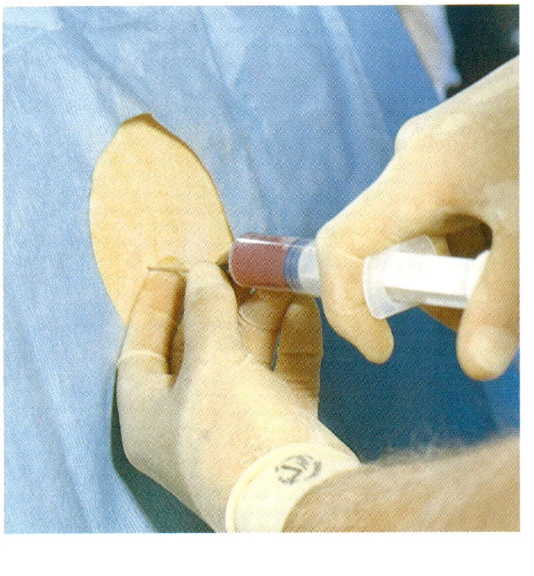

Neurological damage

Epidural block can be followed by neurological deficit, though the incidence of this is extremely rare. There are several causes of neurological sequelae which may be temporary or permanent (Table 6:11).

Trauma

Trauma is probably the commonest cause and usually involves a single spinal nerve. The needle or catheter can enter a nerve and if an injection is made directly into that nerve then some disruption of the fibres can occur. This may lead to a degree of neuritis which can last for some weeks or months. In such cases the patient will usually complain of pain during insertion of the needle or catheter and at the start of the injection. When the block has worn off, the patient may complain of paraesthesia in the distribution of the nerve concerned, with a partial loss of sensation and occasionally some motor weakness. These symptoms and signs usually disappear within a few days or weeks but occasionally last much longer.

Adhesive arachnoiditis

Adhesive arachnoiditis is a serious condition and may result in permanent loss of spinal cord function. It usually follows the injection of an irritant solution and several compounds have been implicated, such as detergent used for cleaning syringes. The local anaesthetic chloroprocaine was involved in several cases in which large quantities were injected by mistake into the subarachnoid space. These reports were followed by animal studies claiming to show spinal cord damage following chloroprocaine injected intrathecally. Other animal data failed to confirm this, and many authorities are still advocating the use of the drug (see p. 154). The accidental injection of a substance other than a local anaesthetic or opioid should, of course, never occur, but unfortunately it does. Substances so injected have included potassium chloride, calcium chloride (in mistake for sodium chloride), thiopental, and even agents for intravenous feeding.

Table 6:11
Summary of Various Types of Neurological Damage Following Epidural Blockade

Pathology	Cause	Onset	Clinical Features	Outcome
Spinal Nerve Neuropathy	Trauma (needle, catheter, injection)	0-2 days	Pain during insertion of needle or catheter. Pain on injection. Parasthesia, pain and numbness over distribution of spinal nerve.	Recovery 1-12 weeks.
Anterior Spinal Artery Sydrome	Arteriosclerosis hypotension	Immediate	Postoperative painless paraplegia.	Painless paraplegia
Adhesive Arachnoiditis	Irritant injectate	0-7 days	Pain on injection. Variable degree of neurological deficit. Often progressive with pain and paraplegia.	May progress to severe disability with pain and paralysis.
Space Occupying Lesion (haematoma or abscess)	Hypocoagulation Bacteraemia	0-2 days	Severe backache postoperatively with progressive paraplegia.	Requires immediate surgery otherwise paraplegia.

Anterior spinal artery syndrome

Anterior spinal artery syndrome is a condition caused by failure of the blood supply in the distribution of the artery. It causes an infarct of the spinal cord with resultant permanent paraplegia. The blood supply of the cord is somewhat tenuous. The anterior spinal artery, though it receives anterior radicular arteries at each vertebra, derives its main supply from the artery of Adamkiewicz (see p. 21). Failure of this supply may occur during aortic clamping or excessive retraction of the aorta during surgery. Atherosclerosis can also cause a diminished blood flow, which may become inadequate with arterial hypotension. Induced hypotension has been blamed for the condition but hypotension by itself is an excessively rare cause of spinal cord infarction. The use of solutions containing epinephrine has been suggested as a possible cause, and high concentrations of epinephrine have caused cord damage in experimental animals. However, in the doses used clinically this would seem to be an unlikely cause of infarction.

The epidural space being a closed compartment, it is possible that infarction could follow the development of excessive pressure within the space. If this pressure were to exceed arterial pressure for more than a few minutes, a permanent lesion could result.

Space occupying lesions

Space occupying lesions such as haematomata, abscesses and tumours can press upon the spinal cord and cause serious cord damage. It is quite common to traumatise a vein during the course of an epidural block. This, however, will not lead to a large and dangerous haematoma in the absence of a clotting defect, which in itself is a contra-indication to an epidural block. Patients given large doses of heparin to anticoagulate them during surgery could be at theoretical risk, though this should be most unlikely if the needle or catheter were inserted more than 20-30 min before the heparin was injected. The use of "mini-dose" heparin to prevent postoperative deep venous thrombosis is held by some to contraindicate an epidural block. Others, however, have reported many thousands of cases without incident. If there is any doubt in an individual patient, a clotting screen can be done to ensure that the heparin has not made the blood excessively hypocoagulable.

Epidural abscesses have been reported following epidural block and are thought to be due to bacteraemia with colonisation of an epidural haematoma. In most cases the patient was suffering from a pyrexial disease. The injection of contaminated material into the epidural space appears to be amazingly rare. That epidural blocks are performed with full sterile precautions and that local anaesthetics themselves are bacteriostatic may account for this. Spinal tumours can, of course, cause paraplegia by direct pressure, but their presence may not be suspected until full neurological recovery fails after epidural block.

If persistant painful backache appears or the nerve block does not fully recover in the expected time, the possibility of a space occupying lesion should be entertained as laminectomy may become urgent if permanent damage is to be prevented.

Catheter problems

The insertion of plastic catheters into the epidural space is usually simple and safe. However, from time to time difficulties arise. The possibility of the catheter entering a vein or the subarachnoid space has already been mentioned. Usually this occurs at the initial insertion, but cases have been reported of apparent migration of the catheter, e.g. the first few injections give a normal epidural block and then a further injection causes a high subarachnoid block. Given the physical nature of the plastic catheter and the toughness of the dura, migration would appear most unlikely. Many of these cases, however, can be explained by the design of the catheter, in particular those with multiple holes. It is quite possible for the distal hole to be in the subarachnoid space (or a vein) while the proximal holes are in the epidural space. As there is a positive pressure in the subarachnoid space it is easier for injected drug to escape through the holes in the epidural space, especially if a slow injection is given (Fig. 6:25a). A forceful and rapid injection will lead to much more drug leaving the distal hole into the subarachnoid space (Fig. 6:25b). Thus there is a good case for using a catheter with a single hole.

Catheters have been known to break during removal and care must be taken if resistance to removal is encountered. Most cases have occurred when an attempt has been made to withdraw the catheter through the epidural needle, the sharp end of which can shear off the catheter end. If placement of the catheter in the epidural space is uncertain, the needle and the catheter should be simultaneously withdrawn. Should a catheter break, leaving a segment in the patient's back, there is no reason to remove it surgically, given the non-irritant

Fig. 6:25 Diagram of a multihole catheter with the distal hole in the subarachnoid space and the proximal holes in the epidural space. a. Slow (low pressure) injection delivers fluid into the epidural space. b. Fast (high pressure) injection delivers fluid into the subarachnoid space.

1. Subarachnoid space
2. Dura mater
3. Epidural space
4. Ligamentum flavum

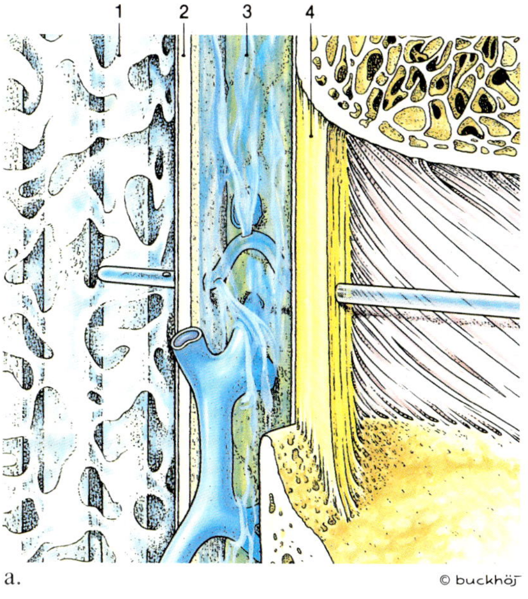

a.

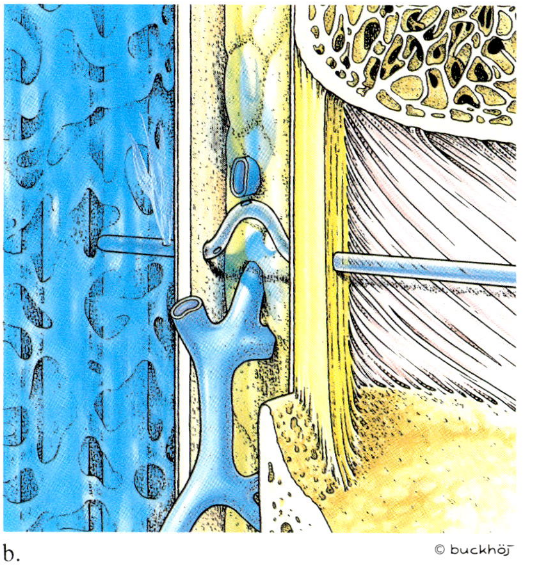

b.

property of the plastic employed. However, it is best to inform the patient and give reassurance that it is most unlikely to give rise to any ill-effects.

If too much catheter is pushed into the epidural space then the behaviour of the catheter is unpredictable. There have been cases where the catheter has encircled a spinal nerve, giving rise to severe pain on attempted removal and the possibility of nerve damage. There is no need to insert more than 3-5 cm into the epidural space in the average patient.

Occasionally it will be found impossible to inject down a catheter. This is due either to kinking or to a clot forming in the catheter. The former will usually respond to a change in the patient's position or withdrawal of 1 cm or so of catheter. If the obstruction is due to a clot, there is no solution except to remove the catheter and insert another.

Summary

This list of complications may appear to be formidable and could deter some from this most useful anaesthetic technique. However, the great majority of mishaps are either preventable, or easy to treat, or both. Much depends on the anaesthetist. He should not only be aware of the complications, he should also be able to diagnose the problem and have a well-ordered plan for treatment. If this sounds obvious, or even platitudinous, nevertheless delay in diagnosis or panic during treatment are important contributors to a serious outcome. A quiet, calm and competent approach is of inestimable value in ensuring patient safety.

References & Bibliography

Albright, G.A. (1979). Cardiac arrest following regional anesthesia with etidocaine or bupivacaine. Anesthesiology 51:285.

Aldrete, J.A. and Johnson, D.A. (1970). Evaluation of intracutaneous testing for investigation of allergy to local anesthetic agents. Anesth. Analg. 49:173.

Aldrete, J.A. and O'Higgins, J.W. (1971). Evaluation of patients with history of allergy to local anesthetic drugs. Southern Med. J. 64:1118.

Benowitz, N.L. (1974). Clinical applications of the pharmacokinetics of lidocaine. Cardiovasc. Clin. 6:77

Blair, M.R. (1975). Cardiovascular pharmacology of local anaesthetics. Brit. J. Anaesth. 47:247.

Boyes, R.N. (1975). A review of the metabolism of amide local anaesthetic agents. Brit. J. Anaesth. 47:225.

Bonica, J.J., Berges, P.U. and Morikawa, K. (1970). Circulatory effects of peridural block. I. Effects of levels of analgesia and dose of lidocaine. Anesthesiology, 33, 619.

Braid, D.P. and Scott, D.B. (1965). The systemic absorption of local analgesic drugs. Brit. J. Anaesth. 37:394.

Braid, D.P. and Scott, D.B. (1966). Effect of adrenaline on the systemic absorption of local anaesthetic drugs. Acta Anaesth. Scandinav. (Suppl) 23:334.

Bromage, P.R. (1978). Epidural Analgesia (complications). Saunders Co., Philadelphia p. 654.

Bromage, P.R. (1980). Epidural narcotics for postoperative analgesia. Anesth. Analg. 59:473.

Bromage, P.R. (1982). Nonrespiratory side effects of epidural morphine. Anesth. Analg. 61:490.

Camporesi, E.M. and Nielsen, C.H. (1983). Ventilatory CO_2 sensitivity after intravenous and epidural morphine in volunteers. Anesth. Analg. 62:663.

Collingsworth, K.A., Strong, J.M., Atkinson, Jr., A.K., Winkle, R.A., Perlroth, F. and Harrison, D.C. (1975). Pharmacokinetics and metabolism of lidocaine in patients with renal failure. Clin. Pharmacol. Ther. 18:59.

deJong, J.A. and Bonin, J.D. (1980). Deaths from local anesthetic-induced convulsions in mice. Anesth. Analg. 59:401.

deJong, R.H., Ronfeld, R.A. and DeRosa, R.A. (1982). Cardiovascular effects of convulsant and supraconvulsant doses of amide local anesthetics. Anesth. Analg. 61:3.

Denson, D., Coyle, D., Thompson, G. and Myers, J.A. (1984). $Alpha_1$-acid glycoprotein and albumin in human serum bupivacaine binding. Clin. Pharmacol. Ther. 35:409.

Denson, D.D., Coyle, D.E., Thompson, G.A., Santos, D., Turner, P.A., Myers, J.A. and Knapp, R. (1984). Bupivacaine protein binding in the term parturient: effects of lactic acidosis. Clin. Pharmacol. Ther. 35:702.

DiFazio, C.A. and Brown, R.E. (1972). Lidocaine metabolism in normal and phenobarbital pretreated dogs. Anesthesiology 36:238.

DiGiovanni, A.J. & Dunbar, B.S. (1970). Epidural injections of autologous blood for postlumbar puncture headache. Anesth. Anala. 49, 258.

DiGiovanni, A.J. (1971). Inadvertent intraosseous injection - a hazard of caudal anesthesia. Anesthesiology 34:92

Edde, R.R. and Deutsch, S. (1977). Cardiac arrest after interscalene brachial plexus block. Anesth. Analg. 55:446.

Englesson, S. (1973). The influence of acid-base changes on central nervous system toxicity of local anesthetic agents. Acta Univ. Upsaliensis, (Dissertation, Uppsala Faculty of Medicine) 166.

Feely, J., Wilkinson G.R., McAllister, C.B. and Wood, A.J.J. (1982). Increased toxicity and reduced clearance of lidocaine by cimetidine. Ann. Int. Med. 96. 592.

Feldman, H.S., Covino, B.M. and Sage, D.J. (1982). Direct chronotropic and inotropic effects of local anesthetic agents in isolated guinea pig atria. Reg. Anesth. 7:149.

Foldes, F.F., Davidson, G.M., Duncalf, D. and Kuwabara, S. (1965). The intravenous toxicity of local anesthetic agents in man. Clin. Pharmacol. Ther. 6:328.

Gettes, L.S. (1981). Physiology and pharmacology of antiarrhythmic drugs. Hosp. Pract. 16:89.

Gissen, A.J., Datta, S. and Lambert, D.H. (1984). The chloroprocaine controversy, I. A hypothesis to explain the neural complications of chloroprocaine epidural. Reg. Anesth. (in press).

Gissen, A.J., Datta, S. and Lambert, D.H. (1984). The chloroprocaine controversy, II. Is chloroprocaine neurotoxic? Reg. Anesth. (in press).

Goolkasian, D.L., Slaughter, R.L., Edwards, D.J. and Lalka, D. (1983). Displacement of lidocaine from serum alpha $_1$-acid glycoprotein binding sites by basic drugs. Eur. J. Clin. Pharmacol. 25:413.

Greenblatt, D.J., Sellers, E.M. and Schrader, R.I.(1972). Drug disposition in old age. New Engl. J. Med. 306:1081.

Gustafson, L.L. (1982). Adverse effects of extradural and intrathecal opiates: report of a nationwide survey in Sweden. Brit. J. Anaesth. 54:479.

Hartley, M. (1975). The strange case of the inadvertent spinal. Br. J. Anaesth. 47, 420.

Kafer, E.R. (1983). Biphasic depression of ventilatory responses to CO_2 following epidural morphine. Anesthesiology 58:418.

Keenaghan, J.B. and Boyes, R.N. (1972). The tissue distribution, metabolism and excretion of lidocaine in rats, guinea pigs, dogs and man. J. Pharmacol. Exp. Ther. 180:454.

Kotelko, D.M., Shnider, S.M., Dailey, P.A., Brizgys, R., Levinson, G., Shapiro, W.A., Koike, M., Rosen, M.A. (1984). Bupivacaine-induced cardiac arrhythmias in sheep. Anesthesiology 60:10.

Liu, P., Feldman, H.S., Covino, B.M., Giasi, R. and Covino, B.G. (1982). Acute cardiovascular toxicity of procaine, chloroprocaine and tetracaine in anesthetized ventilated dogs. Reg. Anesth. 7:14.

Liu, P., Feldman, H.S., Covino, B.M., Giasi, R. and Covino, B.G. (1982). Acute cardiovascular toxicity of intravenous amide local anesthetics in anesthetized ventilated dogs. Anesth. Analg. 61:317.

Liu, P.L., Feldman, H.S., Giasi, R., Patterson, M.K. and Covino, B.G. (1983). Comparative CNS toxicity of lidocaine, etidocaine, bupivacaine and tetracaine in awake dogs following rapid IV administration. Anesth. Analg. 62:375.

Lund, P.C. and Cwik, J.C. (1965). Propitocaine (Citanest) and methemoglobinemia. Anesthesiology 26:569.

Lund, P.C., Bush, D.F. and Covino, B.G. (1975). Determinants of etidocaine concentration in the blood. Anesthesiology 42:497.

Löfström, J.B., Alm, B., Bertler, A., Jorfeldt, L., Lewis, D. and Post, C. (1978). Lung uptake of lidocaine. Acta Anaesth. Scand. (Suppl) 70:80.

Löfström, J.B. (1978). Tissue distribution of local anaesthetics with special reference to the lung. Int. Anesthesiol. Clin. 16:53.

Mather, L.E. and Tucker, G.T. (1978) Pharmacokinetics and biotransformation of local anesthetics. Int. Anesthesiol. Clinc. 16:23.

Mayumi, T., Dohi, S. and Takahashi, T. (1983). Plasma concentrations of lidocaine associated with cervical, thoracic, and lumbar epidural anesthesia. Anesth. Analg. 62:578.

McCarthy, G.S. (1976). The effect of thoracic extradural analgesia on pulmonary gas distribution, functional residual capacity and airway closure. Brit. J. Anaesth. 48. 243.

Meffin, P., Long, G.J. and Thomas, J. (1973). Clearance and metabolism of mepivacaine in the human neonate. Clin. Pharmacol. Ther. 14:218.

Mihaly, G.W., Moore, R.G., Thomas, J. Triggs, E.J., Thomas, D. and Shanks, C.H. (1978). The pharmacokinetics and metabolism of the anilide local anaesthetics in neonates. I. Lignocaine. Eur. J. Pharmacol. 13:143.

Morishima, H.O., Finster, M., Pederson, H., Fukunaga, A., Ronfeld, R.A., Vassallo, H.G. and Covino, B.G. (1979). Pharmacokinetics of lidocaine in fetal and neonatal lambs and adult sheep. Anesthesiology 50:431.

Morishima, H.O., Pederson, J., Finster, M., Sakuma, K., Bruce, S.L., Gutsche, B.B., Stark, R.I. and Covino, B.G. (1981). Toxicity of lidocaine in adult, newborn, and fetal sheep. Anesthesiology 55:57.

Morishima, H.O., Pederson, H., Finster, M., Feldman, H.S. and Covino, B.G. (1982). Is etidocaine more cardiotoxic than lidocaine? Anesthesiology 57:A401.

Morishima, H.O., Pederson, H., Finster, M., Tsuji, A., Hiraoka, H., Feldman, H.S., Arthur, G.R., Covino, B.G. (1983). Is bupivacaine more cardiotoxic than lidocaine? Anesthesiology 59:A409.

Munson, E.S., Tucker, W.K., Ausinsch, B. And Malagodi, H.(1975). Etidocaine, bupivacaine, and lidocaine seizure thresholds in monkeys. Anesthesiology 42:471.

Nation, R.L., Triggs, E.J. and Selig, M. (1977). Lignocaine kinetics in cardiac patients and aged subjects. Brit. J. Clin. Pharmacol. 4:439.

Ochs, H.R., Carstens, G. and Greenblatt, D.J. (1980). Reduction in lidocaine clearance during continuous infusion and by coadministration of propranolol. New Engl. J. Med. 303:373.

Ostheimer, G.W., Palahniuk, R.J. and Shnider, S.M. (1974). Epidural blood patch for postlumbar headache. Anesthesoilogy 41, 307.

Post, C. (1979). Studies on the pharmcokinetic function of the lung with special reference to lidocaine. Acta Pharmacol. Toxicol. 44:1.

Prentiss, J.E. (1979). Cardiac arrest following caudal anesthesia. Anesthesiology 50:51.

Ravindran, R.S., Bond, V.K., Tasch, M.D., Gupta, C.D., Luerssen, T.G. (1980). Prolonged neural blockade following regional analgesia with 2-chloroprocaine. Anesth. Analg. 59:447.

Ravindran, R.S., Turner, M.S., Muller, I. (1982). Neurological effects of subarachnoid administration of 2-chloroprocaine-CE, bupivacaine and low pH normal saline in dogs. Anesth. Analg. 61:279.

Reisner, L.S., Hochman, B.N., Plumer, M.H. (1980). Persistent neurologic deficit and adhesive arachnoiditis following intrathecal 2-chloroprocaine injection. Anesth. Analg. 59:452.

Rosen, M.A., Baysinger, C.L., Shnider, S.M., Dailey, P.A., Norton, M., Curtis, J.D., Collins, W., Davis, R.L. (1983). Evaluation of neurotoxicity after subarachnoid injection of large volumes of local anesthetic solutions. Anesth. Analg. 62:802.

Sage, D., Feldman, H., Arthur, G.R. and Covino, B.G. (1983). Cardiovascular effects of lidocaine and bupivacaine in the awake dog. Anesthesiology 59:A210.

Scott, D.B., Jebson, P.J.R., Braid, D.P., Örtengren, B. and Frisch, P. (1972). Factors affecting plasma levels of lignocaine and prilocaine. Brit. J. Anaesth. 44:1040.

Scott, D.B., Jebson, P.J.R. and Boyes, R.N. (1973). Pharmacokinetic study of the local anaesthetics bupivacaine (Marcain) and etidocinae (Duranest) in Brit J. Anaesth. 45:1010.

Scott, D.B., Owen, J.A. and Richmond, J. (1964). Methemoglobinemia due to prilocaine. The Lancet 2:728.

Scott, D.B. (1975). Evaluation of the toxicity of local anaesthetic agents on man. Brit. J. Anaesth. 47:56.

Scott, D.B. (1981). Toxicity caused by local anaesthetic drugs. Brit. J. Anaesth. 53:553.

Scott, D.B. (1982). Cardiovascular effects of lumbar epidural and spinal anesthesia. Regional Aneithesia. 7 (Suppl.), 521.

Sorel L. Legeunne R. (1955). Modifications de l'EEG du lapin sons l'action de divers succedanes de la cocaine injectes par voie intraveineuse. Arch Int. Pharmacodyn Ther 102:314-334.

Stephen, G.W., Lees, M.M. & Scott, D.B. (1969). Cardiovascular effects of epidural block combined with general anaesthesia. Br. J. Anaesth. 41, 993.

Tucker, G.T. and Mather, L.E. (1975). Pharmacokinetics of local anaesthetic agents. Brit. J. Anaesth. (Suppl) 47:213.

Tucker, G.T., Moore, D.C., Bridenbaugh, P.O., Bridenbaugh, L.D. and Thompson, G.E. (1972). Systemic absorption of mepivacaine in commonly used regional block procedures. Anesthesiology 37:277.

Tucker, G.T., Moore, D.C., Bridenbaugh, P.O., Bridenbaugh, L.D. and Thompson, G.E. (1972). Systemic absorption of mepivacaine in commonly used regional block procedures. Anesthesiology 37:277.

Usubiaga, J.E. (1975). Neurological complications following epidural analgesia. Int. Anaesth. Clin. 13(2):19,50.

Wagman, I.H., deJong, R.H. and Prince, D.A. (1968). Effects of lidocaine on spontaneous cortical and subcortical electrical activity: production of seizure discharges. Arch. Neurol. 18:277.

Wang, B.C., Spiedholz, N.I., Hillman, D.E. and Turndorf, H. 81982). Subarachnoid sodium bisulfite (the antioxidant in Nesacaine) causes chronic neurological deficit. Anesthesiology 57:A194.

Ward, C.F., Osborne, R., Benumof, J.L. and Saidman, L.J. (1978). A Hazard of double-orifice epidural catheter. Anesthesiology 48, 362.

Williams, R.L., Blaschke, T.F., Meffin, P.J., Melmon, K.L. and Rowland, M. (1976). Influence of viral hepatitis on the disposition of two compounds with high hepatic clearance: Lidocaine and indocyanine green. Clin. Pharmacol. Ther. 20:290.

Drug nomenclature

Throughout this book we have used the World Health Organisation's International Non-proprietary Name (I.N.N.) convention. The alternative names of the various drugs, whether proprietary or generic are given in this table.

I.N.N	Other
Local Anaesthetics	
Bupivacaine	Marcaine, Sensorcaine, Carbostesin
Chloroprocaine	2-chlorprocaine, Nesacaine
Etidocaine	Duranest
Lidocaine	Lignocaine, Xylocaine
Mepivacaine	Carbocaine
Prilocaine	Citanest
Procaine	Novocaine
Tetracaine	Amethocaine, Anethaine Pontocaine, Pantocaine
Vasopressors & Sympathomimetics	
Epinephrine	Adrenaline
Ephedrine	–
Isoproterenol	Isoprenaline, Isuprel
Methoxamine	Vasoxine, Vasoxyl
Norepinephrine	Noradrenaline, Levophed
Phenylephrine	Neosynephrine
Opioids	
Fentanyl	Sublimaze
Hydromorphone	Dilaudid
Methadone	Amidone, Phenodone Physeptone, Dolophine
Morphine	–
Naloxone	Narcan
Pethidine	Meperidine, Demerol Dolantin
Other Drugs	
Chlormethiazole	Heminevrine, Hemineurine
Diazepam	Valium
Methacholine	Mecholyl
Midazolam	Hypnovel
Oxytocin	Syntocinon, Syntometrine Uteracon
Temazepam	Normison, Euhypros
Thiopental	Pentothal, Thiopentone

Index

M

N

O

P

R

S

T

U

V

W